HYGIENE
SUPERSTAR

MIKE CZUBIAK, DDS
AND STEVE SPERRY

Copyright © 2019
By Mike Czubiak and Steve Sperry

All rights reserved. This book or any portion thereof may not be reproduced or used in any manner whatsoever without the express written permission of the publisher except for the use of brief quotations in a book review.

Printed in the United States of America
Second Printing, 2019

ISBN 978-0-9968240-1-9

The information contained within this book is strictly for educational purposes. If you wish to apply ideas contained in this book, you are taking full responsibility for your actions. Although the author and publisher have made every effort to ensure that the information in this book was correct at press time, the author and publisher do not assume and hereby disclaim any liability to any party for any loss, damage, or disruption caused by errors or omissions, whether such errors or omissions result from negligence, accident, or any other cause.

www.HygieneSuperstar.com

To our dads

Table of Contents

Hop On!	1
Is It Working?	17
The Science	33
It's a Team Sport	51
Use Your Words	63
Your Helpers	87
For What You're Worth	119
For Your Dentist	141

Foreword

Steve Sperry and Dr. Mike Czubiak wrote this book because they love dentistry, they love health, and they realize that the future of a healthy America rests in the hands of dental hygienists.

Together they bring both a clinical and a personal perspective to a subject that is literally near and dear to their hearts. Coach Steve has been helping dental practices thrive and become wonderful places to work for many years. He has been in thousands of dental offices and he knows people. Dr. Mike is a practicing general dentist who has grown a robust and healthy preventive hygiene practice. He is dedicated to creating an environment that allows hygienists to grow both professionally and personally. He knows hygiene.

Coach Steve and Dr. Mike take turns bringing their experience to the pages of this book in hopes that it will illuminate the importance of the dental hygienist in our practices, in our industry, and in the nation's healthcare system.

What If?

By Coach Steve

What if you could change history? What if the average lifespan of Americans was 120 years? What if the health of every individual you met improved dramatically? What if you had the power to change lives? To save lives? What if YOU were valued higher than a medical MD?

This book is the tell-all, say-all, truth about your impact on human health. We now know that oral health, cascading infection, and inflammation are the root causes of many of the symptoms and diseases that unhealthy patients experience.

What if the demand for periodontal health was greater than exercise, diet, sleep, and second only to drinking water? What would happen to you? What would happen to your practice? What would happen to our industry?

Every significant change in human health started with some sort of a movement. When the pain of poor health outweighs apathy, change occurs. Did you know animal health and wellness is more progressive than human care? Medical doctors can be baffled by variance in therapy. Why do some patients respond differently than others? What is the common thread? What is the link between success and failure?

Hygienists are the solution to a healthier lifestyle. Hygienists are the solution to a more joyful existence. Yes, you, the HYGIENIST.

Section One
HOP ON!
by Dr. Mike

Do the best you can until you know better. Then when you know better, do better.

– **Maya Angelou**

Saving a Life

On a Tuesday morning before our first patient, Cass, my hygienist, came busting into my office. She was excited, anxious, and scared–all at the same time. Cass wanted to show me what she had found. She slapped the report on my desk and said, "We need to save her life."

Lynn is an active 46-year-old mother of three high schoolers. When Cass saw her as a new patient she marveled at how Lynn balanced her work life and home life, while still taking care of herself. Physically she seemed to be in great shape, but her periodontal health told Cass a different story. Lynn had pretty good home care. According to her, she brushed twice a day and flossed religiously, which was her way of saying that she flossed once a week on Sundays. But her upper anteriors, her social six, were surrounded by gingiva that looked decently healthy, so Lynn was not really that concerned with her oral health. She felt satisfied with them but she knew that she should still probably come in and get her teeth checked, since "You know, it's been a while."

Cass took off her loupes, gloves, and mask and sat Lynn up. Throughout the mouth, Cass had discovered moderate to severe periodontitis with bleeding on probing. Cass was sure of this, but unfortunately, Lynn was unconvinced. "My gums bleed, but everyone in my family has bleeding gums. We are just bleeders". Cass inquired about her family history. "I'm not sure if my parents had gum disease. My Mom died of a heart attack at 52 and my Dad doesn't have any teeth."

Thirty seconds later, Lynn was spitting into a vial to be sent to a laboratory for bacterial DNA analysis. The analysis will show if specific pathogenic bacteria are present in her mouth. The excitement and anticipation of the results started as soon as the sample was sent out and lasted the entire week until the results were in, and they were now in.

I picked up the report and there it was. Fusobacterium nucleatum, Porphyromonas gingivalis, and Actinobacillus actinomycetemcomitans, present in quantities that not only put her at risk for periodontal disease but can also be fatal. This means that she has a high risk of following in her parent's footsteps. Scary results to be sure, but Cass was right. She CAN save her life. Cass is a Hygiene Superstar!

Superstar

Just like her peers, Cass is a skilled and well-trained dental hygienist. Caring, thorough and conscientious. But what makes her a Superstar? She is open to new ideas, she thinks about what she does and why, she embraces science, she looks to improve and stay on the cutting edge, and she has the courage to break new ground. She…is in the game.

Cass doesn't see herself as part of the hygiene department and she doesn't see herself as being the one that just "cleans" her patient's teeth. She sees herself as a part of the patient's medical healthcare team, integrated as a partner in the patient's overall health. She understands the link, the missing link in many practices, between the oral and systemic health of her patients. I mean, really understands. Many dental professionals will certainly say the mouth is the window to your health, floss or die, healthy mouth, healthy body, blah, blah, blah. But do they really believe it? Do they really understand it? Do they really educate their patients to it?

Thinking about bleeding gums, deep pockets, furcations and mobility from the traditional perspective of periodontal disease do not lend itself very well to thinking about its systemic effects. The idea that the main goal of periodontal maintenance is smooth roots and no deposits is outdated by science. Instead, a hygiene superstar sees the mouth as somewhat of a petri dish, growing and disseminating pathogens that can then go and cause both periodontal and systemic disease. This new more modern perspective is about the pathogens and the resulting inflammatory response. So it is important to realize that the control of this petri dish, the oral cavity, is critical in reducing pathogens that are responsible for destroying the periodontium as well as causing chronic disease and death. A study illustrated this systemic effect when it showed that with an increase in the population of the bacteria P. gingivalis, heart attack and stroke risk doubles, and when the population of these dangerous critters gets even bigger, the risk can quadruple.

This book is all about this missing link. Sure, you have some great clinical skills, but do you know what you really need to know, and do what you really need to do in order to save your patients' lives? This knowledge is a prerequisite to becoming a Hygiene Superstar.

Inflammation-The Missing Link

Inflammation is the missing link that is crucial to understanding why an unhealthy mouth can lead to an unhealthy body. Chronic inflammation is a root cause of so many chronic diseases like heart disease, strokes, diabetes, and periodontal disease, just to name a few.

Yes, chronic inflammation is the enemy and it has been studied and shown to be responsible for all of these diseases and more. Treating people with these chronic diseases accounts for 75% of our nation's more than $2 trillion of health care spending. Even though chronic diseases are mostly preventable, they are still responsible for 70% of the deaths in the United States. We do have our work cut out for us and you are right in the middle of it. You are so, so important.

Inflammation is a natural defensive process that has great health benefits. When you get a cut, your body is set up to heal that cut, and it does that by going through the process of a inflammatory response to resolve the problem. An inflammatory response is also triggered by bacteria in your mouth. But too much for too long puts a great burden on our defenses. This is referred to as inflammatory burden. Day in and day out, these oral bacteria cause chronic inflammation and the release of proteases and reactive oxygen species. This results in tissue damage that in the mouth we see it as attachment loss and bone loss, but in the body, we see it as the destruction of other tissues like the endothelium of blood vessels, intestinal linings and elsewhere.

The inflammatory products damage tissue by breaking the tissue down and making it more porous. In the mouth, this leads to porosity in the sulcular gingiva that then allows periodontal pathogens and the inflammatory products themselves to pass into the tissue and consequently into the vascular system.

When a patient has a chronic inflammatory bacterial condition in their mouth the inflammatory process never turns off. Their body never gets the opportunity to rest. This increase in the inflammatory burden is just too much for the body to handle and the body gets sick.

This inflammatory burden is killing people and it needs to stop. Steve and I are committed to the fight. Will you join us?

The Movement

"Complete Health Dentistry" has started, but most dentists and dental hygienists have never even heard of it. The movement is made up of progressive medical and dental professionals(Superstars) that are passionate about preventing disease, not just treating the result of the disease. They focus not just on the oral cavity, but on the whole body. They know that so much death and disability are caused by inflammation, and as it turns out, the mouth is a huge source of that inflammation. Hundreds of studies have shown that periodontal disease is a root cause of systemic inflammation. No longer can the body be divided up between our medical and dental communities. We are all in this together. We need to be united, we need to work as one.

Complete Health Dentistry is about seizing the opportunity to create better lives, to change lives, to save lives. We are very fortunate to be in the position that dentistry affords us. We see our patients frequently, we build up great relationships with them, we gain their trust, and we care about them. This puts us in a very special spot to not only screen for oral diseases but also systemic disease. This is especially true since most of our patients see us much more often than they see their very own physician. We can become their "oral physician" and screen them for head and neck cancer, hypertension, sleep disturbances, airway issues, pH issues, and more.

We can educate our patients on nutrition, fitness, smoking cessation, and even more.

You can see that there are many facets to Complete Health Dentistry. This book will cover the "blood-borne" subset. This subset is about oral pathogens, mostly coming from our periodontal pockets, wreaking havoc on our oral and systemic health. Gaining knowledge of this connection and how to more effectively control our dangerous oral pathogens is just the beginning. We can grow our understanding of how lifestyle, genetics, and diseases affect our systemic health, and we can screen for these health risk factors also. Screening can be done by simply asking the right questions, doing the right tests, or by simple observation. This information will allow us to incorporate individual risk factors into our treatment plans. This will help us achieve optimal oral health much more effectively. This will also initiate conversations to help our patients make changes in their lifestyles and seek referrals to other healthcare workers.

Reading this book gives you the opportunity to get in early, and be the Paul Revere of Complete Health Dentistry. It is time. What is the message that we want to spread? Mouths matter! We need to know this, understand this, and communicate this to make a difference. And what a difference it can make.

Better oral health leads to better overall health and a better quality of life. This is true, but the word needs to get out. It is not okay to keep it as the best kept secret anymore. Be the messenger. It's easy, just start talking about it. I've found that people are fascinated by it. You'll find that the oral/systemic connection is way more fun to talk about and way better received than talking about the need to floss so you don't get gum disease. And, it won't feel like nagging to either you or the patient. Just saving lives!

Why People Die

You have probably heard stories of people passing a treadmill stress test at their cardiologist's office and then dropping dead two days later. Or a story about someone fit and "healthy" like Jim Fixx, who wrote the "bible" on running, but had a massive heart attack and died at the age of 52. These may seem like medical mysteries or just plain bad luck, but are they?

Take, for instance, a treadmill test. You pass that, and boy, you feel great. A clean bill of cardiovascular health, right? Many would be surprised to know that passing the test only tells them that their coronary arteries are less than 70% blocked. That sounds good unless you know another statistic: 86% of heart attacks occur in people with a less than 70% blockage!

Heart disease is the number one killer in the United States. There are many facts that aren't common knowledge like they should be. Heart attacks are not just for men; they are also the number one killer of women. Yet, due to gender bias, they are often under-diagnosed because even physicians think of it as a man's disease.

My mother was at the movies a few years back. She started to feel "not good." It felt like an elephant was standing on her back. She had had pain shooting down her left arm for three days. She wanted to just lay down and rest but my stepdad said, "No, you are going to the hospital." He calls me and I rush down to the emergency room and there she was, sweating, ashen skin tone, and denying the possibility of having a heart attack. She had all the symptoms of a heart attack including denial. I hear her tell the ER team that her pain in her left arm was because she had just gotten a new bra and it was probably just a bit tight, and the chest pains were from too much Diet Coke. Really Mom?!? At the time, I was so impressed by the crew that night. They kept my mom calm by going along with her about not having a heart attack. But it wasn't until the next morning that I found out that they hadn't called in a cardiologist because they weren't sure she had had one! Any man would have been diagnosed as he was coming through the doors!

The under-diagnosis of heart disease in women is a serious problem. To make things worse, for 40% of women who have a heart attack, their first symptom of heart disease is a heart attack.

Recent studies show that up to 50% of heart attacks are triggered by oral infections. What is killing people is inflammation. Bacteria elicit an inflammatory response from the body. This response leads to a great deal of destruction: from the breakdown of the bone that supports teeth to the piercing of a woman's uterus, which causes preterm or stillborn births. Over 12% of pregnancies in the United States end with a preterm birth (less than 37 weeks). Periodontal disease makes a woman seven times more likely to have a preterm birth. Recent medical studies have shown that the oral cavity is the breeding ground for and the source of the bacteria Fusobacterium nucleatum (Fn) found in the amniotic fluid of the placenta. Besides being a major constituent of dental plaque and a cause of periodontal disease, Fn gets into the bloodstream, goes into the uterus, and makes the uterine lining permeable. This allows other bacteria to leak through, causing infection and inflammation which can result in premature birth or even death.

A good reason to be a Hygiene Superstar?

Shift in Thinking

In school, I remember hearing the hygiene instructor lead the class in what was almost like a cultish chant. Delivered with the call and response enthusiasm usually reserved for a high school football game, our instructor shouted repeatedly:

What's the most important piece of calculus to remove?

On cue, without hesitation, as trained, the whole class would say:

The last one!!!!!

These words rattled through the caverns of my soul for decades, holding me to a goal that I had accepted, until I realized that it was wrong. Now, during scaling and root planing or a maintenance visit, we must focus on reducing pathogenic bacteria. Of course, deplaquing and deposit removal is still important, but the goal has totally changed. And success is not measured by lack of bone loss, but by eradicating inflammation. You've probably had one of those patients with bright red, puffy, bleeding gums but not a lot of deposits. What's going on? Inflammation! And going only after deposits and telling the patient to floss more just isn't enough. It just doesn't work. I think we have all been there.

There are also patients like Lynn who present pretty well visually. Then, about two probing sites into the charting you realize that looks can be deceiving. It's like opening up a dam. You know that in a few minutes you're going to be elbow deep into a bloody prophy. Cass sees this as an opportunity. An opportunity to fight this silent killer. Cass knew that she was the one to possibly save Lynn's life.

Hygiene Superstar

Section Two
IS IT WORKING?
by Dr. Mike

I think it's very important to have a feedback loop, where you're constantly thinking about what you've done and how you could be doing it better.

— **Elon Musk**

Really???

Let's take a moment to reflect on what you do right now. How does what you do work for you? Do you fully understand why some patients have such great results while others...not so good? For me, I had too many patients that I just wished would do more. I didn't know that there was more that I could do. I went through the motions, while in my heart I knew that whatever I was doing was not enough.

Hi Mr. Gross, nice to see you again. You may remember that I had recommended a three-month interval for your maintenance and I see that it has been six months.

I thought you were on board with that. I remember walking you up to the front and requesting that they set you up with a three-month interval.

Oh, your insurance won't cover it... You say you've been taking really good care of yourself?... Brushing twice a day, flossing almost every day, do you get any bleeding when you...no, OK, OK. Let's take a look.

When was the last time you brushed your teeth?... Just before coming here today...OK, when did you last eat a ham sandwich?... A couple days ago, OK, OK, let me just get an additional mask.

You marked on our form that you would like to talk about lightening your teeth, so, like something in a lighter green? Are you concerned with your breath at all, Mr. Gross?...Do I smell something? Well, I am assuming it is your breath but I can check for any dead animals in the operatory.

Let me just put down a drop cloth and we will get started.

Why would patients choose to neglect themselves? Why is change so hard? Although you probably can't reach everyone, dedication and education will fuel your passion, and passion will improve your success rate with all of your patients, even those like Mr. Gross.

Bloody Prophys

We all have patients who think that bleeding in the mouth is normal, they say, "I always bleed." But if they were brushing their hair and their scalp started to bleed, do you think they would be concerned? Obviously, that would be cause for concern. What if they went to their MD and she wasn't concerned? Maybe it isn't bleeding as much as it did last year. We are doing better, right? No. Scalps shouldn't bleed, neither should gums.

For adults, the area of gingival tissue is about the same area as the palm of your hand. And like your hand, it has epithelium on the outside acting as a protective surface armor. When we see bleeding on probing we know that the armor has been pierced and the sulcus is harboring bacterial pathogens that are infiltrating into the tissue and then into the bloodstream. Sulcular gingiva is literally being bathed in a pathogenic marinade of toxic bacteria. Needless to say, the gingiva, the bone, and the patient's whole body don't like this.

Our traditional protocol is to scale the area, instruct the patient to floss more, and maybe have a patient use an oral rinse like Listerine or Peridex. We may even place an antibiotic locally in the pocket. We do all of this and usually, we find that it works sometimes, but other times it doesn't get much better. Hopefully at this point, the patient confesses to skipping a day of flossing, otherwise, we feel that we have failed them. A sense of helplessness may overcome you so you bring the dentist in, and the dentist says, "You should floss more." Fast-forward three, four, or six months, and they are back. We dig in and whammo, still bleeding. So we go in for the kill, "Tell me, ma'am, did you skip even one day of flossing?" Dang it, she's been totally diligent. She's even developed calluses on her index fingers. We are definitely missing something.

If we were just concentrating on bone loss, some of these patients would get a pass. Probably because we didn't look at the beginning signs of bone loss presenting itself on our bitewing radiographs as a slight rounding or breakdown of the interproximal lamina dura. Out of sight, out of mind. We'll check it out next time. "Did I mention, make sure you floss more?"

Double Masking

When I first started in dentistry, wearing a pair of latex gloves was offensive. It was perceived as an insult like the dentist was afraid of catching something from the patient. And truth be told, we did tend to put them on only if we had a "feeling," or if someone just seemed infectious. HIV in the mid-80's changed that. Our lack of understanding about the routes of transmission made it really easy to start gloving up and masking up. I liked wearing a mask. No longer did it bother me if a patient had just polished off a plate of spaghetti marinara right before their appointment. Nor did it matter if I had done the same.

But by donning masks, we inadvertently took away one of our age-old diagnostic tools, our nose. Our sense of smell has been very useful in medicine for centuries. In the emergency room, it works well for recognizing diabetic ketoacidosis; on the battlefield, gas gangrene; and in our operatories, periodontal disease. Another one is alcohol ketoacidosis, whose smell has been described as that of nail polish remover and results from heavy alcohol consumption. A lifestyle clue to say the least

Periodontal disease has a very distinct smell. It is different than the run of the mill "morning breath." Malodor comes from volatile sulfur compounds (VSC) that are produced by bacteria breaking down proteins that mainly reside in the periodontal pockets and on the dorsum of the tongue. The makeup of the bacteria will alter the composition of the VSCs to give it its own unique smell. Think rotting fish or rotten eggs.

In the past, when I would see patients who complained about bad breath, I would look around and hope that I would find a big piece of chicken stuck between #30 and #31, or a nice perio abscess distal to #18. When I didn't, I would assume that it was coming from somewhere besides the oral cavity. It is true that VSCs can originate from extra-oral sites due to chronic sinusitis, nasal inflammation, post-nasal drip, diabetes mellitus, cirrhosis, liver insufficiency, uremia, trimethylaminuria, or lung carcinoma. But in a study examining hundreds of patients with bad breath, 87% of them originated from oral causes.

They also found that VSCs increased with the number, depth, and bleeding tendency of periodontal pockets. One of the VSC compounds is hydrogen sulfide, which is found in infected periodontal pockets. The levels of this compound have been found to be higher than the levels needed to damage epithelial cells. It also can increase the permeability of the oral mucosa and disturb the body's defense against bacterial infections.

In other words, bad breath is a sign that bad things are happening. This shouldn't be ignored and we shouldn't be so quick to blame it on something other than periodontal disease. I know sometimes you might be tempted to double mask for some of the worst offenders, but really, pull your mask(s) down and smell.

The Petri Dish

There are 500-1000 different types of bacteria that make up the human oral flora. Most of these actually benefit us and prevent disease. But some of the bacteria in our mouths are quite harmful. Each tooth surface can contain anywhere from one thousand to one billion bacteria per tooth surface. In fact, a quantity of saliva equal to the size of a nickel contains over 8 billion bacteria, more than all the humans on the Earth.

I compare our mouth to a petri dish because, like a petri dish made to optimally grow bacteria, our mouth is also pretty much optimal for bacterial growth. The mouth provides an ideal place to grow bacteria because unlike the other tissues in or on our bodies, the hard surfaces in the mouth don't desquamate. They don't shed like skin or intestinal linings. This allows them to attach to those surfaces and grow and grow, creating destructive dental plaque. Although saliva helps bacteria by providing protein nutrients to them, the main job of saliva is to wash away these microorganisms. This is why xerostomia (dry mouth) leads to such rampant bacteria growth.

For the harmful bacteria, their ability to do harm grows as they come together to form biofilms. At first bacterial cells are deposited onto a surface from the saliva, and they arrange themselves into clusters. They begin to produce a gooey matrix made up of all sorts of microorganisms like fungi and algae, along with debris and corrosion products. This matrix is held together by sugary molecular strands called extracellular polymeric substances (EPS). These strands allow the bacteria colonies to develop complex three dimensional, resilient, well-protected communities called biofilm. The biofilm then releases small or large clumps of cells to attach to another surface or to another biofilm, so it can continue to grow and infect other sites.

It is very important to acknowledge the fact that periodontal pathogens can be spread from site to site or person to person. You've probably seen that patient with the worst inflamed gingiva you've ever seen, only to meet their spouse who has the same exact inflamed gingiva. Using a bacterial saliva test, you can analyze the bacterial type and quantity in the saliva, and you will see that both people will have very similar oral floras. And for you dog lovers, yes, you may be swapping pathogens with Fido, too!

The good news is that we are pretty good at killing off bacteria, but the bad news is that we currently aren't doing a good job controlling bacterial biofilm. That gooey matrix makes biofilm very resistant to most mouthwashes, antibiotics, and even scaling. Alone, a bacterium is vulnerable and easily destroyed. But let it grow and mature into a biofilm, and that gooey matrix held together by EPSs creates a slimy coating that acts like a tough, defensive shield over the colonies and protects them from destruction.

Six-Month Recalls

You may have heard the story about the birth of the six-month recall interval. It was a big win for preventive dentistry in a world where people previously only saw a dentist for emergency procedures. But all these years later, we should educate our patients to follow science instead of a marketing campaign.

It all started back in the 1930s. The ad men from Pepsodent Tooth Powder needed a catchy line. They had landed a sponsorship on the hugely popular radio show *Amos and Andy*. At this point in history, people were not very preventative-minded and dentists, well, they did a lot of extractions. The ad men came up with, "Use Pepsodent twice a day. See your dentist twice a year." Later, they changed it to, "For the safety of your smile… use Pepsodent twice a day…and see your dentist twice a year."

This was the dawn of the 6-month interval, propelled by pop culture in the '30s and burnished into our psyche when the program landed on television in the '50s. It is unclear whether the ad men pulled the number out of the air, or if they were referencing the father of modern dentistry, Dr. Pierre Fauchard, who wrote in 1728:

Those who are diligent on the conservation of their teeth and who wish to avoid being the victim of their error or their negligence ought to have them examined two or three times every year by an experienced dentist...

Hopefully, it came from science through Dr. Fauchard and onto the *Amos and Andy* show. But things have changed since 1728. We now have to consider our modern view of pathogen reduction. Studies show that biofilm takes about 90-120 days to reach its potential to wreak havoc on our periodontium. After that, our risk for heart attack, stroke, cancer, diabetes, etc. goes way up. If our patients are on a six-month interval, they are potentially poisoning their bodes with pathogens that originated in the mouth. You will find some patients that do great with a six-month cycle, but that number will usually be rather small. Remember, our criteria is not buildup, but rather inflammation, so "great" means inflammation-free. The majority of patients should find themselves on a three or four-month cycle. We don't need to find much buildup on these patients to recommend these shorter intervals, just inflammation.

Yes, our patients will have to be retrained. It has been deeply ingrained into the American psyche to think that twice a year is sufficient. Insurance companies pay twice a year so that proves it, right? It's awesome that some insurance companies are getting it and allowing payment for three or four "cleanings" a year. It's a perceived truth that will take some effort to change, but it will be worth it, and if a patient values their health and wellness, it will be a slam dunk. If not, don't give up. After they hear the message enough, they will get it. Patients don't do what they need, they do what they want. The facts are compelling, and the truth is undeniable, so give them a reason to want it.

It Will Never be the Same Again

Understanding the real enemy makes it easier to understand the clinical presentation of our patients, whether they are teenagers with gingivitis, adults with other health risks, or elderly people with poor hygiene. This knowledge will assist the Hygiene Superstar in making smart, confident clinical decisions. Additionally, with the knowledge that these biofilm infections lead to systemic inflammation and therefore systemic disease, our Hygiene Superstar is well prepared to educate his or her patient to a level that would otherwise not have been realized.

Can you see the potential? Annually, heart disease alone kills about 630,000 people per year and costs the U.S. $200 billion. We can make a huge impact. We WILL make a huge impact!

Hygiene Superstar

Section Three
The Science
by Dr. Mike

Science and everyday life cannot and should not be separated.

– Rosalind Franklin

Science by the Numbers

Superstars or not, we are doing a pretty good job of saving lives. It has been shown in studies that people do much better when they receive treatment for their periodontal disease. Even coming from the perspective of traditional periodontal treatment, this should not be a real surprise. Reducing bacterial pathogens, even if not done as efficiently and effectively as possible will lead to better overall health.

> **FACT: Treatment for periodontal disease is associated with a significantly reduced overall risk of cancer.**
>
> **FACT: Treatment for periodontal disease leads to improved glycemic control in type 2 diabetic patients for at least three months.**
>
> **FACT: Intensive periodontal treatment reduces systemic inflammatory markers and systolic blood pressure and improves lipid profiles.**

Reducing systemic inflammatory markers, that's what hygienists are doing right now. We now know that this inflammation reduction is a direct result of decreasing the quantity of pathogenic oral bacteria like P. gingivalis, A. actinomycetemcomitans, P. intermedia, T. forsythia, T. denticola, F. nucleatum. and many others.

Proliferating and thriving in the mouths of most Americans, these bad guys are instrumental in creating chronic disease that ends up costing us plenty. 75% of our healthcare expenses are put towards treating chronic illnesses like heart disease, strokes, and diabetes!

In 2016, a paper published in the Postgraduate Medical Journal showed that there are three major mechanisms that periodontal pathogens use to cause arterial disease. They presented Level A (highest quality) evidence proving that periodontal disease causes cardiovascular disease. The take-home message was "The dental community has a substantial opportunity to mitigate the number one cause of morbidity and mortality, namely cardiovascular disease, by elucidating feasible effective management of periodontal disease due to high-risk pathogens."

We know now that when we treat a patient's periodontal disease, we are improving a patient's cardiovascular health as well. That is proven. Other associations, like P. gingivalis and rheumatoid arthritis, may be proven false in the future. That's fine. At worse, we are reducing our patients' risk of dying from the world's biggest killer and at best we are reducing the risk of suffering from Alzheimer's, cancer, diabetes, preterm birth, and many other inflammation-based diseases.

Learn more by checking references.
HygieneSuperstar.com/references

Heart Disease and Strokes

FACT: Every single day, heart disease and strokes kill about 2200 Americans.

FACT: In the US, every 40 seconds someone has a stroke and every 4 minutes someone dies from it.

Heart disease kills ten times more women than breast cancer. It is the number one killer of women. In fact, each year, more women die from cardiovascular causes than do men, yet it is still thought of as a man's disease. These women are often completely unaware that they are at risk for heart disease. You might think that our current medical screening tests would help us be more proactive, but no. Just as in dentistry, coming out of school with an out-dated understanding of periodontal disease, physicians are operating with an antiquated view of cardiovascular disease.

A common myth is that heart attacks and strokes are caused by plaque building up inside blood vessels like grease in a sink's drainpipe growing until the blood flow is obstructed causing a heart attack or stroke. But, researchers have shown that it is not plaque that causes a blockage that triggers a heart attack or stroke, it is a blood clot. What happens is that plaque builds up inside an arterial wall and when inflammation is present, the artery lining can tear open exposing the plaque. The body does its best to seal this tear by forming a blood clot. It is this blood clot that can abruptly cause a blockage, halting blood flow and leading to a heart attack if it blocks a coronary artery or a stroke if it blocks the flow of blood through an artery supplying the brain.

FACT: Strokes are the 3rd leading killer of people worldwide causing the death of over 5 million people each year.

FACT: Nearly 2/3 of all fatal strokes occur in women.

FACT: 45% of heart attacks and 33% of strokes happen in people under 65 year of age.

Research shows that periodontitis increases the number of pathogenic bacteria leading to an increase in systemic inflammation which doubles our patients' risk of heart attack and stroke. Research has shown that as periodontal inflammation increases, so does the inflammation in the carotid arteries and when it decreases in the mouth, it also does in the carotids. Studies like this have led the American Heart Association to publish their conclusion that there is overwhelming, unequivocal evidence that periodontal disease is independently associated with arterial disease. What they are saying is that periodontal disease is a root cause of arterial disease.

Diabetes

FACT: Diabetics are 4 times more likely to have a heart attack or stroke than non-diabetics.

Don't think that your patients are safe because they are only pre-diabetic. They still have three times the risk of having a heart attack or stroke. And with periodontal disease, the relationship with diabetes is bi-directional, in that the presence of one disease tends to promote the other, and that the meticulous management of either will help the treatment of the other. Uncontrolled periodontal disease makes controlling blood sugar levels very difficult just as uncontrolled blood sugar levels make periodontal disease very hard to manage. Great diabetic control and great periodontal health are crucial.

With diabetes, your body doesn't make enough insulin or it can't use its own insulin as well as it is supposed to. We eat food so that it can be turned into sugar (glucose) for our body to use for energy. Insulin is a hormone that is made in the pancreas and is used to help transport sugar into our cells. When insulin is not able to do this, sugar builds up in the blood. This puts stress on the blood vessels, causing them to get injured more easily. This can lead to heart disease, kidney failure, blindness, and lower-extremity amputations.

Another complication of diabetes is that it hinders

white blood cells' ability to fight off infection. Diabetes causes blood vessels to thicken, which slows the flow of nutrients to and waste products from body tissues. When this happens, the body has a harder time fighting off infection. Since periodontal disease is a bacterial infection, diabetics can have an escalation of periodontitis and gingivitis (gum inflammation).

FACT: In 2012, 29.1 million people (almost 10% of all Americans) had diabetes.

FACT: The percentage of Americans age 65 and older with diabetes is over 25%.

FACT: Diabetes was the 7th leading cause of death in the United States in 2010, causing 69,071 deaths and contributing to 234,051 more deaths.

Cancer

FACT: Periodontal pathogens P. gingivalis and F. nucleatum have a role in cancer development and progression.

We are just starting to understand how the periodontal pathogens growing in our pockets affect the growth of cancers throughout our body. Colorectal cancer and pancreatic cancer are two that have been studied recently. Researchers have found that F. nucleatum grows in the periodontal pockets, leaches into the bloodstream, breaks through the epithelial lining of a distant site like the colon, and inhibits our body's own natural tumor-suppressing cells. This leaves us much more at risk of developing a tumor.

When a patient develops periodontal disease, their risk for cancer goes up. They are growing these bad pathogens and putting their whole body at risk. If we can improve their oral health, their risk goes down, and they are much more apt to stay alive.

FACT: Men with periodontal disease have a 63% higher chance of developing pancreatic cancer than those without it.

FACT: Risk for head and neck cancer increases up to five times when periodontal disease is present.

Oral HPV infection has emerged as a risk factor for head and neck squamous cell carcinoma. It has been shown that chronic periodontitis may facilitate the acquisition and persistence of the Oral HPV infection. This may be through direct toxic effects of the periodontal bacteria and their products, and/or through indirect effects of the inflammation that they cause.

The effects of periodontal disease on oral cancer have been investigated in many studies. These studies have shown that there is a 2–5 fold increase in the risk of oral cancer among patients with periodontal disease as compared to those without periodontal disease.

The results of studies on periodontal disease and cancer vary widely due to the complexity of cancer genesis. The variation in risk assessment will continue until more understanding of the process is revealed. What is widely seen in the studies is that we may decrease the risk of cancer in our patients by reducing F. nucleatum and P. gingivalis in our patients' mouths. That is something that a hygiene superstar can definitely do!

What Else?

Researchers are busy at work checking out all sorts of possible systemic consequences of inflammation. Some of these consequences are just quality of life issues, but others are fatal.

FACT: Chronic periodontitis was found to have a high association with erectile dysfunction in adults young and old.

FACT: Dentate individuals who reported not brushing their teeth daily had 22 to 65% greater risk of dementia than those who brushed three times a day.

FACT: P. gingivalis accelerates abdominal aortic aneurysms.

California researchers tracked 5611 seniors for 17 years and found that never brushing at night boosted the risk for death during the study period by 20-25% compared to brushing every night. Never flossing lifted mortality risk by 39% vs daily flossing. Not seeing a dentist in the previous twelve months raised their risk of death by up to 50% compared to getting dental care two or more times per year.

FACT: One major predictor of early death was missing teeth, even after other risk factors were taken into account.

Dr. Bradley Bale and Dr. Amy Doneen run heart attack and stroke prevention clinics. They are very progressive and very successful in preventing cardiovascular disease by recognizing the importance of inflammation. They have written a profoundly important book called *Beat the Heart Attack Gene*. You need to read this book. They are huge believers in you, the hygiene superstar.

FACT: From the Bale/Doneen method of heart attack and stroke prevention, the first action step is to take care of your teeth.

Learn more about the Bale/Doneen Method and the book *Beat the Heart Attack Gene*.
HygieneSuperstar.com/baledoneen

Dental Education Not Keeping Up With Dentistry

Like an astronaut coming back from an intergalactic space voyage, Lauren was about to be bombarded with questions. I couldn't wait to hear the news from our newest dental hygienist, fresh out of hygiene school. Tell me the state of the art. Wow me with the latest. I've been out of school for over 30 years, so what a great opportunity to find out how far the field has evolved in the last quarter of a century. So we sit down and as if I am in a trance, the words just pass through my lips, "tell me..."

What I hear from this astronaut is that all the stressed-out aliens are tooling down overcrowded roads in 1985 Honda Civics, reaching down to grab another Elton John tape to jam into the car stereo. And no, the cars don't levitate or run on nuclear fission, they are gasoline-powered, pollution emitting jalopies. In other words, nothing had changed. How can that be? So I ask Lauren, "What's the most important piece of calculus to remove?" You guessed it. She said proudly, "The very last one." Ugh!

Really, I shouldn't have been surprised. Dentistry is both an art and a science. The science part is, of course ,the vast reservoir of knowledge gained from years, and centuries of carefully planned and executed studies. This is where dental education shines, once the highest standard of proof exists, they are all in. The art part is using individual clinical experience to affect judgment. Maybe a bit more emotional or "hunchy" but nonetheless a valuable aspect of every experienced clinician. This is much more difficult to teach, and also more difficult to justify when defending your curriculum. To make things worse, the trend towards Evidence-based Dentistry may hinder the creativity that research and practice has always enjoyed.

The American Dental Association defines Evidence-based Dentistry as "an approach to oral healthcare that requires the judicious integration of systematic assessments of clinically relevant scientific evidence, relating to the patient's oral and medical condition and history, with the dentist's clinical expertise and the patient's treatment needs and preferences." What that is supposed to mean is that decision making comes from the intersection of clinical judgment, patient needs and wants, and the most current relevant scientific evidence. The problem with this is that so often, the scientific evidence lags behind clinical impressions and experience. The best studies are longitudinal studies, studies that track people over many, many years. The results arrive excruciatingly slowly, and if we wait until we obtain consensus from multiple longitudinal studies, we would never be using so many of the wonderful restorative materials or preventive products that we use today. How does your latest prophy paste stack up against pumice over the next two decades? Is it more harmful to the teeth, are there longterm benefits, is it worth the extra patient expense? Most clinicians will say yes, new formulations with exciting ingredients like calcium phosphate are very promising and worth using now!

Can we wait to implement new, more modern, efficient, and effective hygiene techniques and procedures, as well as ground-breaking new products that can lead to saving peoples lives? Do we want to wait?

Be a Pioneer

Thousands of years ago, Ancient Egyptians used dried myrtle leaves to treat muscle pain. Somewhere around 400 b.c., Hippocrates, the father of modern medicine, prescribed willow bark tea for the pain of childbirth. In 1758, the Reverend Edward Stone of Chipping Norton, Oxfordshire, chewed a twig of white willow to ease his pain and fever and was so impressed with its effect that he wrote to the Royal Society in 1763 to alert them to its benefits. What was it about these plants that made them so effective in treating pain and fever? When chemists analyzed willows in the 1800s, they discovered that they contained salicylic acid, the basis of the modern drug aspirin. The point here is that these people were pioneers of pain management. They were clinical researchers. They were observers. They tried a promising plant remedy and relied on their own clinical results to push ahead this important development that added to the quality of life for countless people. A trend I have seen in dentistry in the last few decades is a switch from clinicians counting on their own observations to relying solely on research from universities and manufacturers. A trend that has some merit in certain cases, with the complexity of our new modern materials, but is sure to slow down the advancement of our field in general.

I bought a diode laser about twelve years ago. I started doing things with it, I started cutting. I did frenectomies, fibroma removals, gingival recontouring, almost anything that I might have used a scalpel for. But then, I heard someone talking about how the energy from the laser could kill off bacteria in the periodontal pockets. I searched for current, relevant evidence to support this use of a laser in every journal that I could find, and nothing! So, I started my own clinical trials. I would use it on some patients, in some areas, first in pockets that were unresponsive to my traditional "tricks," and then to other less severe pockets and lo and behold, I saw some really good results. I liked what I saw. Reduction of gingival inflammation, bleeding points, and tenderness. I discussed my observations with periodontists in my area and I got nothing. No excitement, no curiosity. If you are into periodontal disease reduction, why wouldn't this get you excited? Two words: no studies.

Recent studies have demonstrated that the Waterpik® oral irrigator is superior to dental floss in reducing bleeding and as effective in reducing plaque. A study at the University of Southern California found that a three-second treatment of pulsating water at medium pressure removed 99.9% of plaque biofilm from treated areas. My mom has been using a Waterpik since the 60s and she loves it, swears by it. So has her son, the dentist, been recommending it? No, I waited until 2009 (47 years after it was invented) to recommend it because that is when the studies came out. It's a wonder that I am not waking up at night thinking about all of the biofilm that was not removed because my patients were not using Waterpiks until 2009.

As you get older, you get a different perspective on life, including your professional life, and you notice that you acquire more confidence. You can speed up this process by learning more, observing more, thinking more. Pick up your journals, participate in online hygiene groups, attend classes, partner up with your dentist to create your own clinical trials. Do it, be like my mom, be a pioneer.

Hygiene Superstar

Section Four
It's A Team Sport

by Coach Steve

There doesn't have to be any one hero.
There just has to be a whole lot of
heroes working together.

– Stephanie Lodding, RDH

In The Middle of It

The military calls the first line the "spear" of the attack. The marines typically are the spear. We are the marines in healthcare. We have the opportunity to lead. We are being asked to lead. Will we answer the challenge? Will we be the ones? We can be. We should be.

Being influential is such a gift. You have spent so much time developing relationships with your patients and getting them to trust and respect you. No one on their healthcare team has the same relationship that you have with them. You see them two, three, or four times a year. You talk to them, care for them, educate them. Now, you can take that relationship and make it even more valuable by expanding what you look for, what you talk to them about, what you care about, and what you educate them on. And the word will get out. The public is smarter than we imagine. Consumers are being forced to know about their own health. I love technology for this reason. Everyone is seven questions away to better health. The answers all point back to YOU. Does that excite you? It excites me…

What does the future of healthcare look like? Do you see hygienists being right in the middle of it? I do. We are the influencers. We are the educators of the future. We have the studies. We have the tests to determine risk factors. We have the questions to ask. We are the answer to better, more sustainable health.

Getting Everyone on Board

It starts with a big vision! How is it that young men and women go marching off to war? Putting themselves in harm's way. Why do they do it? What motivates them? If you ask them, they will most likely tell you the same thing. They believe in what they are doing. They believe in the cause. They believe in the mission. They like being a part of something bigger than themselves. How about you? Is saving lives a good enough reason? A reason that "puts fuel in the tank" for the journey? Working for money will get you so far, but in order to really cover some ground, you need more fuel and being a part of something bigger is just that.

How about the front office, the assistants, the other hygienists? Will they come aboard? Is the vision compelling enough to get these soldiers to join you in the battle against unnecessary suffering in the hands of chronic disease? Your vision, your passion, that's what's going to help get them to join you. They will also need to be educated. Practice bringing up the oral/systemic conversation. Try out your knowledge and see how it goes over with your team. I see this all the time. Teams get totally excited about this. They will care, just as you do. They will want this.

It takes a team to do great things which include the

doctor/owner. Are they on board? Why wouldn't they be? Change can be hard, especially if it looks like more work for them. They will need to buy into the vision. They will need training. If you can get your doctor to the point of asking how then we are already there. Believe it or not, the hard part is getting your doctor to that point. The easy part is moving forward. The owner will need guidance. The good news is help is out there.

Will everyone be on board or will Debbie Downer try to throw a wet blanket on everything? There is a good chance that you may have someone that isn't jumping up to wave the banner of Complete Health Dentistry. That's OK. They may feel that everything is just fine as it is, they fear change. Many people have fear of the unknown, so know that these team members may just need additional time, knowledge or encouragement. We can deal with that.

Assembling the Right Team

We know we can't go alone. We need that superstar team. I wish I had better news but I don't. The team that brought us this far may not (almost always will not) be the team that takes us to the next level. Who cares and who is just picking up a paycheck? The team determines how far we go. You can try to influence and change others, but in my experience, that is the hard way. Recruiting or growing the superstar team is a big part of the battle. The good news is that the people we are looking for are looking for us. We want to attract the winners. The ones that see the vision. That want to do better. The ones that see the future. Yep, we need the superstar team and we need to constantly look for the passionate ones. The ones like us.

The team has to be our focus. The weakest link on the team can hold the rest of the team back. We all need to buy into the same vision. Never stop looking to improve your team.

It is vitally important to get the right people on the bus but even more important to help those that aren't going to our destination off of our bus. But for most dentists, this very important task is the scariest thing that they will ever do. Dentists like to please people, they are relationship people. Their team is like family. How do you get an underperforming family member off of the bus? Very few dentists are good at this. I have taught this skill to hundreds of dentists and have heard over and over again that it is the single most important management skill that they have ever learned. It is the first step to assembling that superstar team.

You need to champion the cause to find awesome team members. Everyone needs to see the vision and commit to it. If they don't, fine. Everyone will be better off with them changing buses. If your doctor has problems with getting people off of the bus, help by supporting their decision and encouraging them to take action. And if they just can't, have them get some help.

Leading

I had great parents. They always told me to act like you own the place. I take that skill everywhere. I may not be anyone, but I will act like I am. Just because you don't own the place doesn't mean you can't act like the owner. And in a way, you do own the place. I think you do. You are the practice. This is your home. It is your time to lead. Leading is paramount to accomplishing your vision.

It's your vision and now, it should be the practice's vision. It has to be. Leadership is learned and everyone can learn to lead. You are the leader in this task. You are more important than the doctor. YOU are the change agent. You change lives and save lives.

Leading your team is so important. Yes, I said it. Your team. This is your team, right? Of course! Then let's lead it. The good news is that you've already done step one of being a leader- having a compelling vision. Done. Next, you will need to move people to action. But be careful, how you do this is critical. If you take the dictator approach, you will fail. No one likes it, no one responds well to this. Don't be that person! A better is to encourage people to help find solutions. How can we best implement Complete Health Dentistry into our practice? Embrace ideas, consider all suggestions. Don't squash others, empower them. Allow them to grow.

The team is looking to you to help them feel a part of the movement. Empower them to feel purpose and to participate in the vision. You can use logic. You can use belief. You can use passion. You can educate. You can walk the walk and talk the talk. You will need all of this and a bag of chips to align the team to our new model. The good news is that your team wants hope as well. They want what we are saying. To be more. To follow your passion for helping others.

So, step up and take this leadership position. Maybe it will feel strange to you but this is too important. Don't wait, take the lead. Be the Rudolph and all of the other reindeer will love you!

You Can Create the Change

Later on in this book, we will discuss finding your home. If you cannot affect change, then leave. Is it really worth your time, effort, and energy to be that "change agent?" In some practices, yes. In others, no. Is apathy the reason for lack of growth and progress? How do you become the "change agent?"

Continual learners are continual earners. If you want to be the best, you must learn with the best. The change process begins with unfreezing the current culture. In order to unfreeze anything, the owner must want to change. If you want to go fast, go alone. If you want to go far, go as a team. In his book, *7 habits of highly successful people*, Stephen Covey says that 10% of any organization can change the entire organization. You must have advocates on your team. The doctor must trust you enough to be your biggest advocate. This entire book is all about change. Where do you start? Always start with you.

You can do it. You got this. What can't you do? Really... What can't you do? If it is important to you, YOU will do it. Find a way. Manipulate. Fight. Be a pain. Always ask, when are we going to start saving lives and changing lives? Why are children great at getting what they want? They ask until they get it. Ask and you shall receive. Ask and it will be given to you. We are meant to do this. It is our destiny. It is what we are supposed to do. Join the movement…

Hygiene Superstar

Section Five
USE YOUR WORDS
by Coach Steve

One must be frank to be relevant.

– Corazon Aquino

Communicating a New Concept

When Austrian physicist Ludwig Boltzmann proposed that all matter was composed of atoms and molecules, he met a whole bunch of resistance. Scientists scoffed at the idea. People were not ready for such a novel idea. Well, the good news is that persuading people to take better care of their mouth so that the rest of their body will be healthier is not such a foreign concept. People (including most healthcare workers) have heard that and in their hearts believe it, they just don't know how it all works. The concept of inflammation and inflammation burden is also not totally new, but it will take some thoughtfulness in order for our patients to get it.

Some people will get it just by telling them, hey, if you don't keep your mouth healthy you are going to increase your chances of having a heart attack or stroke or get cancer or diabetes. Others will need some proof, so use an example of how oral health affects something else in simple terms. For example, if you have diabetes and bleeding gums, your risk of premature death increases by 400 to 700 percent. Generally, when you give one example, that example will pacify them and they won't have a difficult time with any other connection. But there will be a few that just don't see it. They are the out of sight, out of mind patients that don't really want to know.

Ignorance is bliss type of people. You know they are out there. They are the ones that go through periodontal therapy and then take the next year off before they come back for their recare visit. These are the challenging ones, but as you get better at communicating (especially listening), the number of these people will diminish. What does it take to get through? Everyone is just a little different.

But doesn't everyone want to live longer, healthier? I know I do. My grandpa on my mother's side lived till 92. The day before he died he rode a horse. I have a picture in my bedroom with his two sons and his dogs. What a stud my grandpa was. I want to live until 120. I have so much to do. I have so much to see. I want to live a HEALTHY long life. I suspect that many others do too. A testament to this is the longevity centers like the Cooper Clinic in Dallas Texas, the Mayo Center in Illinois and the Cleveland Clinic in Cleveland. They combine specialists to gauge and monitor health. They exist to give us that baseline of health, to bring all western medicine together and assess and ameliorate our risk factors. What will kill you? What is that weak link in our physiology? What's the best way to help live longer and healthier lives? See your hygienist.

People are receptive to the concept. We just need to use our knowledge of each individual patient so that we can deliver the message in a way that's easy for the patient to receive. Make sure you use confirmation questions to validate that the message has been understood, "Does that make sense to you? Do you see where I am going with this? How do you feel about that? Does that trouble you?"

Patients don't know what they don't know. How you tell them is the secret. Telling divides asking unites! Ask the question to which the answer is the message... Seriously, this could be the single biggest take away from this book. We have to stop telling patients their problems and start asking questions that relate to them. Do you want to know HOW to get patients to own their problems? Ask questions! It may take a bit longer, but they will own it.

"Seeing that your parents both died from heart attacks, what concerns do you have about your own heart health?"

"Are you interested in keeping your body's inflammation to a minimum?"

"Are you more of a reactive person or someone who likes to benefit from being proactive? Because, as you know, sometimes in health we don't get a chance to react, it is just too late."

There is so much helpful information to be gathered. Do you ask the sleep question? Do you ask the snoring questions? Do you ask the heart disease questions?

Diabetes? Stroke? Do you ask the pregnancy questions? How are your patients from an energy standpoint? Vitality? Do you know their family history? Do you even ask the real questions? When is your check out date? When you are 70? 80? 90? 100? If you could live healthily, how old do you want to live?

Patients need to better understand the importance of dental hygiene. Yep, this is our fault… We have to own this one. The doctor is the key to the recall system. If your doctor does not begin every conversation or end every conversation with, "Does Steve have his continuing care appointment scheduled?", we have stolen some of that importance away from the patient. We, the hygiene department, must train our doctors to do this with ALL patients. They need to do this every day that ends in Y. Y? Because patients only value what is emphasized. The first thing and the last thing out of the doctor's mouth is critical to patients.

Sending a Consistent Message

Do patients ever remember anything that you say just once? OK, well maybe one or two, but most people need to hear the same thing multiple times in order for it to sink in. That's why it is so critical to have a system in place so that one consistent message is being delivered to the patient at any one time. In Dr. Mike's practice, they have seven hygienists. Although they try to schedule the patients with the same hygienist they had before, that just isn't always possible. This isn't a problem since the patient will have a very similar experience no matter which hygienist sees them. Sure, there will be different styles and personalities, but the message is the same.

That's how it is now, but it hasn't always been like that. Many years ago during performance reviews, Dr. Mike heard from several of his hygienists that they were concerned that there was an inconsistency in treatment and education happening within the hygiene department. This led him to do a hygiene-specific coaching program that completely unified their treatment and message. The hygienists loved it and they all knew that they were now speaking the same language.

What about the rest of the office? You got it, they were included in the training so that they too could have the same understanding and be able to communicate intelligently with the hygienists and doctors. Everyone speaking the same language, delivering the same message, emphasizing the same things, that is the sound of a fine orchestra. But, of course, every orchestra needs a conductor. Who do you think that is? You're right. It's you. You will be in charge of making sure the patient, the doctor and the front office are all playing the same tune.

SHO-Time

You use your communication skills to gather information from the patient, to communicate your findings to the patient, and to discuss treatment recommendations with the patient. Then the doctor comes in. You could tell them what is going on with the patient in private, but why lose that opportunity for the patient to hear it again? This is called a hand-off. When done well, it is called a Superstar Hand-off (SHO). Let's talk about "SHO time."

In front of the patient (and I mean literally in front of the patient), fill the doctor in with everything that you know the doctor wants to hear and also everything that you know the patient needs to hear again. Once the doctor leaves, reiterate what the doctor had said and make sure that the patient is on board with whatever was said. You bring your patient up to the front and bingo, another hand-off. This is your time to tell the front office what they need to hear and again, what the patient needs to hear again. Once you leave, the front office will reiterate what you have said and like magic, you will have a patient that knows exactly what is going on and takes responsibility for themselves.

You may have heard the terms blocking and scripting from the acting world. Blocking is where you stand, sit or move. Scripting is what you say. This is important for the hand-off. The blocking and scripting should all be pre-arranged. What, where and how you communicate to the doctor and the front office should be worked out in advance. Practice with them. The doctor may want to hear the results of the medical history update, the oral cancer exam, restorative exam, cosmetic exam, perio exam and the complete health exam (inflammatory risk factors). The front office may want to hear about their recare interval, other treatment needed, number of appointments, duration of appointments, and urgency of the appointments.

Every hand-off, every time, nothing to be left out. It becomes a habit, a very effective habit and the confusion of the patient and team members diminishes. Ask any front office team member if they have ever had a patient at the front desk, after their diagnosis for SRPs, wait until the hygienist and doctor are out of sight, and ask, "What is root planing? Can't I just get my teeth cleaned?" Argh!

Practice hand-offs. Ask for feedback. Did you get all of the information that you needed? Ask and perfect. There is a certain happiness that will come over you when you nail that hand-off. You will be happy, the team will be happy and the patient will be well taken care of. It's SHO-time!

Learn more about hand-offs.
HygieneSuperstar.com/hand-off

Finding Your Schtick

I wish every hygienist could start out by being a server in a restaurant. It's an awesome training ground for developing your schtick. Using your personality, your style, to connect with each patron in a matter of minutes is definitely a skill, a skill that can be developed. The cool thing about the restaurant business is that you get immediate feedback in the form of tips that let you know how you did. If you deliver a phenomenal experience, you will immediately be rewarded. If you fail miserably, then you will see that in your tip also. What a great way to develop your skills.

Every hygienist I've met has a unique style of communicating. A different schtick. Some do it with a nurturing warmth. Some with a playful teasing. Some with a firm directness. Some with a serious concern. Some are great at humor. Some will beat you into submission. Some are laid back. Some talk you to death. What is your style? Is it working for you? Does it work with all of your patients? You are probably seeing where I am going with this. Some styles work for some patients and not others. The goal is to have a style, a schtick that is comfortable for you but, most importantly, is effective for most of your patients. For the other patients, they may need a different schtick.

Unfortunately, a common style that I see hygienists

use is also probably the least effective one. It is the shame, "You let me down" style. Because hygienists understand the importance of good home care, they have the tendency to convey their disappointment which leads to guilt and embarrassment. How many patients don't show up for their appointments because they don't want to be yelled at? Did they ever get yelled at? No, but it felt like that. People can be very sensitive. If you feel like you are nagging, or you respond with a frowny face, or even just a low (non-energetic) tone in your voice, you may have just "yelled" at your patient.

A hygienist friend of mine had a patient in hygiene school that wouldn't do much in the way of home care, and he felt horribly guilty about that. He told her that he would prefer that she hurt him during the cleaning and "yell" at him for not taking care of himself. She thought he was joking, but no, he said that then he would feel like he has gotten his punishment and that would relieve his guilt. Ok, sure she was weirded out for the next couple of cleanings, but then she realized, "I want him to take care of himself." She started to search for a style that would get through to him. And finally, she found it. She turned into the Richard Simmons of hygiene. She was the over-the-top encouraging coach. Rewarding him with praise for even the most minor of improvements. He ate it up and suddenly he wanted to please, anxious for her to see what he had accomplished and really appreciating that she didn't give up on him.

Schtick is not just your style, it is the phrases you use, your facial expressions, your body language, the tone in your voice. I know a hygienist that says, "Oh my gosh!" to everything. A patient would say, "I just picked up some cat food at the market." She would respond, "Oh my gosh!" in a very high (energetic) tone reinforced by a big smile and eyes that are lit up, and it works. People love it. Are you conveying energy, happiness, and joy?

Over your career, a superstar hygienist will develop a really effective schtick with variations depending on the type of patient. Mirroring, reflecting back a patient's own style, is the first place to start. Nurturing warmth may not be the most effective style for a serious engineering type patient. A Type A person probably won't want the long explanation of everything. You start to talk too much and they are likely to stop you and tell you to get to the point. Use fewer words with this patient and take a direct, quick path. Your schtick may be storytelling, "Just last week, I had a patient with a very similar issue with their recession…", but in this case, you need to go the direct route, "Your recession concerns me because…"

Dr. Mike tells me this story:

Nancy, a very serious patient of mine comes in last year and when I ask her if she had any concerns, she said: "Yes, I do." She said, "You're not funny". After watching my "serious face" freeze for a moment, she continued, "all of my friends see you and they all laugh and talk about how funny you are, and I have to be honest, I don't see it." I tend to automatically mirror patients, but now whenever Nancy comes in I have to force myself to be funny even though my natural schtick is to be funny. Her friends are light and fun, and she... she's not. She still responds the best to confident concern when we are discussing health but I have to throw in a couple of zingers just so she doesn't feel left out!

Call it your winning formula. It is different in everyone. Finding your magic is critical. The key to schtick is identifying what works for you.

Using Magic Words

We want to get our patients to optimal health. So why is it so hard to get them to do what we want them to do? And, not just saying yes to us, but really following through. How many promises made to you by your patients have been broken? "Yea, I'm gonna start…" We can try begging and reasoning but mostly we will fail. We don't want our patients to say yes, just to say yes. We need our patients to want it. Being told what to do is getting less and less effective. We are bombarded with so many advertisements and people wanting us to buy insurance or give to their charity that when we hear these requests our brain just shuts them down. That's the bad news, but the good news is that there are some tools that can help open up a patient's mind so that they can be open to new ideas and suggestions. These tools are ordinary words that when used properly, become magical.

If you want to really improve your communication skills both at the office and in your personal life, read the book, *Magic Words* by Tim David. He talks about magic words like "but", "because", and "if", among others, and how important they are in language.

"But" is a powerful word because it minimizes whatever is before it and emphasizes whatever is after it. If a patient asks "Do I need to do X-rays today" and you say, "We would be risking missing active decay in your mouth but we could wait until next visit," all they will hear is, "it can wait until next visit." If you say, "it can wait until next visit, but we would be risking missing active decay in your mouth," they are much more apt to do it today. Who wants active decay in their mouth?

"Because" satisfies our brains need for reasoning. Just like a child, always asking why, our brain needs the "because." In his book, Tim David talks of how years ago, Harvard University psychologist Ellen Langer did a study in which she asked to cut into a line of people waiting to make copies. She politely said, "Excuse me. I have 5 pages. May I use the Xerox machine?" She did this over and over again and found that she was able to cut in 60% of the time. Then she tried it again, this time saying, "Excuse me. I have 5 pages. May I use the Xerox machine because I am in a rush?" By giving a reason she was able to cut in 94% of the time. But, here is where it gets interesting. She did it again, this time saying, "Excuse me. I have 5 pages. May I use the Xerox machine because I need to make copies?" Not even giving a real reason, she was able to cut in 93% of the time. This is why the parent answer, "Because I said so" works. For our patients, instead of just telling a patient to come back in three months for their next visit, at the minimum say, "Let's set you up for your next visit three months from now because that will be the best time to have you back in."

I love the word "if." Used correctly, it quickly opens

up the brain to all sorts of new ideas. "If" is great for getting through creative barriers. Asking Mr. Gross, "What is it going to take to motivate you?" will usually result in an "I don't know." But asking, "If you were really motivated to care for yourself, what would you say would be the reason why?" is much more likely to lead to answers.

The book also highlights the importance of using names to emphasize a point. "I see active infection in your mouth" will make a bit of an impact, but, "Sarah, I see active infection in your mouth" will make a much bigger impact. When people hear their name, their attention gets laser-focused on the message. And, of course, by using their name, you will get the added benefit of making it easier to remember them.

As a general rule, stay positive. Responses of "Great!", Awesome!", or even "Oh my gosh!" will dramatically improve your connection with your patients. Avoid the word "little." It is used too often without realizing that it is totally negating everything that we have already said. "There is a little bleeding on the lower right." Wrong. "Your gums are bleeding on the lower right because you have active periodontal disease." And lastly, get pumped up. Be energetic. You are on stage. It is time to shine, you have lives to save.

Words to eliminate! Top 7 worst words to use in a

treatment presentation...

Little
Watch
Possibly
Maybe
Might
Consider
Think About
Kinda

The worst is when I hear, "There is a little bit of decay we should watch possibly for the future, maybe we might consider thinking about doing." Wow!

Learn more about magic words.
HygieneSuperstar.com/magicwords

Not A Four-Letter Word

Sell. What is your gut reaction when you hear that word? Many hygienists I have met over the years really don't like that word. The reality is, ALL we do is sell. We are in a service business and we sell our services. But don't worry. I have been teaching treatment conversations for over 30 years and I have learned some things along the way. The more you push, persuade, and try to sell, the less dentistry there is to do. This is a common mistake that dentists make. Pressure is put on the hygienists to produce big numbers and to "sell" products and procedures that they don't believe in.

If you are in one of these practices, then you need to talk with the doctor. It is entirely possible that they have not communicated their treatment philosophy with the team or educated the team to the benefits of these products and procedures and, once explained, they may seem perfectly reasonable. If after knowing their treatment philosophy and learning about these products and procedures you still are not comfortable, that may be a good reason to find another home.

When you focus on treatment, the practice will lose. When you focus on long-term care and health, the practice will win. Become unattached to the treatment and very attached to hygiene. When your culture changes to 100% pre-appointing in hygiene, the office will take off. When a patient leaves with an appointment for their continued oral treatment and care they are family. Invite your patients to join your "family." Family is such a strong word. It means something to everyone. When they are family, everything else will work out.

This is not to say that hygienists don't have a role in treatment conversations and case presentations. Asking questions, screening patients, and having conversations about their needs and desires are vitally important to the value of the recare appointment. Let them know that you care, "If I could wave a magic wand and change anything about your mouth and smile, what would you want to see changed?" The responses can be surprising. I heard an 83-year-old woman say that she would change the fillings out on her front teeth because they are making her look old. Fair enough. Why should we allow a couple of simple fillings to make her feel old?

We in dentistry tend to be really good at keeping our services a secret. Most patients don't have a clue about what we have to offer. After offering Invisalign for about 8 years, a practice that I coach added Invisalign to their promotional loop that plays in their waiting room. No joke, 45 minutes later, they had a patient committing to treatment all the while saying, "I never knew you guys did this!"

Back in the '50s, Dr. Mike's Grandpa Joe sold Chevrolet cars. It was an exciting time as the much anticipated Corvette was coming out. When they arrived at the dealerships, they were so popular that everybody wanted to get a look at them. So many that most salesmen didn't pay much attention to any of these potential customers unless they fit the profile of what they thought a Corvette buyer was. They would cherry-pick the "best" customers. By the end of that year, Grandpa Joe was the top Corvette seller in California. People would come from miles around to buy one from him. Parents would be grumbling, "I don't know why my son dragged me all the way over here to buy this car, but he wanted to buy it from you." The reason was easy. He didn't cherry-pick. He would treat everyone as a potential buyer and would let even the young kids sit behind the wheel and get excited about it. Seems simple enough, but it is really easy in dentistry to let our own biases affect who we offer our services to. Offer our services to everyone. Never assume that a patient won't want or can't afford necessary treatment as well as optional treatment. It just isn't fair.

As a superstar, when you talk to your patients about oral/systemic health, you will be happily surprised at what happens with some of your patients. Patients that you couldn't imagine caring about any part of their health will get really motivated and excited by it. Becky, a hygienist from Arizona tells me this story about a hard-headed retired teacher Colleen. Years ago, she had a chronic apical abscess on #31. Didn't hurt at all. Could Becky get her to take care of that? Nope, not for two years. Then Becky started talking about the oral/systemic connection and the increased risk of stroke that she was subjecting her body to. A light went on, most likely due to her family history of stroke, and she was scheduled with the endodontist the very next day. Colleen was so appreciative and she had a higher appreciation for what Becky does. Saving lives, all in a days work!

It's Not a Marriage Without a Commitment

You have spent your time, put in a great effort and now what? Is the patient ready to move forward? Have they had all of their questions answered? Are they committed? During a hygiene check, if a dentist is told that, "We discussed the need for a nightguard," OK, and… Is the patient committed to moving forward with this treatment? A superstar hygienist isn't satisfied with just educating a patient, just talking about stuff, the superstar wants action. To get action, we need a commitment.

Getting a commitment is really easy. All you have to do is ask. I like to use the "Three-Part Closing," otherwise known as the "comfortable close."

Three easy questions:

- Are you comfortable with what we have shared with you?
- Do you understand why you need…
- Do you see any reason why we would not move forward today with treatment?

You run through these questions often enough and

they will just dance off of the tip of your tongue. You will feel more in control because the uncertainty of the patient's acceptance and understanding has been confirmed. And, if you want to see a big smile come from the doctor, this is how you get it. This will save them the time that they would take during the exam, or, worse yet, the time the front office would have to take in order to determine if the patient is committed. Nobody is in a better place to handle obstacles or misunderstandings than you. You know this stuff. Don't leave it up to the front to explain to a patient why they need two "extra" recare appointments per year.

Should you be talking about money? Some doctors and hygienists will say that they can't talk about money because it is too complicated and it isn't professional. Plans all pay at different rates. Benefits vary. These are not good enough reasons in my mind to turn the transaction into a car buying experience. Does anyone like how cars are sold? Sitting you down in a room with someone you don't even know to hear the big price and to be sold add ons? Preface it by telling them that it is just a ballpark number and that the front office can investigate their insurance and give them a more accurate estimate. Wouldn't you want to find out while you were considering your options whether something was 5 dollars, 500 dollars or 5000 dollars? You have probably had one of those patients that you thought was totally committed until they got up to the front and they found out that their copayment was going to be $50.

With that, they back out. If the money had been dealt with in the back, you would have had the opportunity to see that you hadn't created enough value in the patient's mind in order to create the "want" that is truly necessary for a commitment. That is what will help you improve. Asking the right questions and getting a commitment is how action begins.

Section Six
YOUR HELPERS
by Dr. Mike

Never limit yourself because of others' limited imagination; never limit others because of your own limited imagination.

– Mae Jemison

The Fight It Deserves

We've been there before. Armed only with our scalers, curettes, and prophy paste. Backed up by a super-variable version of "home care." And yes, I'm doing air quotes as I say home care. That was pretty much it, maybe a referral card to the periodontist. That was all we had to fight off the most common infectious disease in the world. And you know what, it really never felt like enough. Now with our team of helpers, our modern tools and products, we can give periodontal disease the fight that it deserves. It doesn't take magic, it just takes helpers that will aid you in accomplishing what you know you can do because of your paradigm shift from going after deposits to going after biofilm. From preserving teeth to preserving lives. So, bring your open mind and come meet your helpers.

Ultrasonics

I was at a hygiene lecture recently in Las Vegas listening to a hygiene superstar speak about the Perioscope®. The Perioscope, if you don't know, is an intraoral camera for the periodontal pocket. It is a very small camera that enables a clinician to see right into the pocket. She was showing calculus removal with a Dentsply Cavitron® ultrasonic scaler. There were 190 hygienists in the room sharing in the excitement of seeing chunks of calculus fly off of the root surfaces. They watched as she treated this patient pocket by pocket. Someone asked, "I don't see you using your hand scalers, how often do you pick them up?" The superstar said, "I pick them up every time they roll over and block my ultrasonic. I pick them up to get them out of the way!" There was a noticeable tension that developed and I understood why. We work so hard to master our hand scalers, with their multiple bends and angled cutting surfaces. We take pride in our mastery of fulcrums, intraoral and extraoral. And I have to say, the sound of steel on a smooth root is… like the voice of an angel. Now, she is going to tell us that the same thing can be accomplished in less time and without using every instrument on our tray?

What I learned in school was that ultrasonics were for lazy people, people that didn't want to do a good job.

I believed that, for a good portion of my dental career. What a shift in thinking when I saw the studies that showed that ultrasonics were as good as hand scaling in reducing bleeding and increasing clinical attachment level on single-rooted teeth. On multi-rooted teeth, the advantages of the small tips surpass hand scaling for access into harder to reach areas, especially furcations. And this is based on just going after plaque and calculus deposits. Thinking like a superstar, we are also going after the biofilm, breaking up that gooey matrix, killing off the bacteria and flushing them out.

To accomplish this higher goal, we need to use slimmer ultrasonic tips. I like the Dentsply FSI-SlimLINE inserts (FSI-SLI). They come in right and left and are used in pairs. They are wonderful for getting deeper into the pockets because they are made specifically for each side of the tooth. This allows the power of the tip to not only reach the subgingival deposits but to create an acoustic effect which is bactericidal. Even if we don't find many deposits, it is crucial to spend extra time in the pocket to break up the biofilm and to flush out debris. Your patients will appreciate these tips also since they are used with a lower power setting and compared to hand scalers, there is less tissue trauma. Standard straight inserts work well for supragingival deposits but are not as effective subgingivally as the SlimLINE inserts. Use your ultrasonic scaler as your primary tool and your hand scalers as an adjunct.

When belt-driven handpieces were replaced by air-driven handpieces it changed dentistry. Dentists jumped on it. I am surprised, in light of the evidence dating back to 1979, that the revolution to ultrasonics has taken such a long time. I would think this would be really good news for most hygienists. The ergonomic benefits alone are worth putting down the hand instruments and picking up a power scaler. It is also important to note that most research has been done using more standard inserts. The newer slimLine inserts are designed to be so much more effective, which is why I have seen much better results since making ultrasonics my primary weapon to remove deposits and destroy bacterial biofilm.

Learn more about ultrasonics.
HygieneSuperstar.com/ultrasonics

Lasers

Pop quiz: Name the doctor that made lasers a household name? Yep, you guessed it, Dr. Evil. In the movie Austin Powers, Dr. Evil was going to put a "laser" on the moon to create his "death star." It took me years after that movie came out to stop saying laser the way Dr. Evil said it, "laaay...zer", while of course, doing the necessary air quotes. Sure the FDA approved the first soft tissue laser in 1987, but in good old dentistry fashion, we have been able to keep it a secret for all of these years.

The big breakthrough was in the mid-90s, when diode lasers hit the market in their compact, inexpensive packages. Well, I guess it wasn't a big breakthrough since most dental offices don't have lasers. There are several things that turned some dentists into early adopters of diode lasers. The first was the ability to cut like a scalpel but without the bleeding. Diode lasers use heat to cut soft tissue which also cauterizes the tissue at the same time. Nothing is more disappointing than debanding an orthodontic case, getting excited to see the beautiful results, and seeing the excess gingival tissue that had proliferated cervical to the archwire obscuring half of the facial surfaces of an otherwise beautiful smile. No problem. Topical anesthetic applied to the gingiva and a diode laser will remove the excess tissue as you sculpt around each tooth. Or an operculum on a child creeping over the distal of a lower molar causing pain with each bite. Easy. Three-minute procedure, no pain, no bleeding, that's modern dentistry.

Lasers are high-intensity lights that vary in their abilities depending on the power and frequency of the light that they produce. The sun produces many frequencies of light. Visible light that we see, infrared light that makes us warm, ultraviolet (UV) light that interacts with our melanin and makes us tan, and many others. Each of these abilities is intensified by power. The infrared light that warms you will vaporize you if you get too close to the sun (increasing the power of the sun). Lasers only produce a single frequency depending on the medium that they use. The first lasers in dentistry used CO_2. Then there were ND:YAG lasers that were crystals. Diode lasers use a chip, a semiconductor made of a combination of elements like gallium, aluminum, and arsenide. This produces a frequency that is perfect for soft tissue since it likes to interact with dark things like melanin and hemoglobin. The use of a chip in these lasers has allowed them to be much more affordable and a lot less complicated. This simplicity has also allowed them to be made smaller and smaller which has made them completely portable.

For you, the dental hygienist, the two most common uses of the diode laser is to reduce the bacterial load in the pockets during a maintenance appointment and to remove diseased tissue, granulation tissue, in the pockets during scaling and root planing (SRP) appointments. Laser bacterial reduction (LBR) lowers the bacterial count of gram-negative bacteria from the billions to just hundreds. This reduction will decrease the severity of the bacteremia in the patient and the potential exposure to the hygienist. It has been shown to last for 4-6 weeks, delaying the reformation of sulcular biofilm. When the laser is used in conjunction with SRPs, it is called laser-assisted periodontal therapy (LAPT). Besides just removing diseased tissue, the laser has a bactericidal effect and stimulates fibroblasts for faster regeneration of healthy soft tissue (biomodulation).

Yes, it is a whole new tool and a whole new language creating huge possibilities and you, the hygienist, are on the front line of this revolution. Right now hygienists are reducing bacteria loads, removing diseased tissue, healing aphthous ulcers and herpetic lesions, and desensitizing root surfaces. Get yourself trained and see what a hygiene superstar can do.

Learn more about lasers.
HygieneSuperstar.com/lasers

Oral Rinses

People love mouthwashes and I do too. I really like an oral rinse that can kill off harmful bacteria, not just in the pockets but all over that petri dish we call our mouth, including our tongue, cheeks, palate, and tonsils. But, most people use them for cosmetic reasons, to freshen their breath or to whiten their teeth. Some do use them for their therapeutic effects, caries prevention, and the control of periodontal disease.

There seems to have always been quite a bit of confusion around the use of oral rinses when it comes to helping periodontal health, both in the eyes of the general public and with dental professionals. But, with the popularity of Chlorhexidine (CHX), dentists and hygienists started to really see the value of them. We loved not only the studies that made it the "gold standard" of oral rinses, but also the visual evidence we saw. Sure we liked the improved periodontal health, but the carcasses of dead bacteria staining the teeth a dark green/black, well that was satisfying…until, of course, we had to clean it off. That is just one of the down-sides of CHX. Patients also hate the bad taste, the staining of their tongue and the inability to taste food. It is much more effective against free-floating bacteria as opposed to bacteria encased in biofilm. There may also be a bacterial resistance that can develop so longterm use is not recommended. But even short-term compliance is a big issue. It doesn't matter how great a product is if it sits unused on the sink. So how do the other rinses stack up against the "gold standard"?

Listerine has been very popular, with the essential oils doing a pretty good job supragingivally. Essential oils have been around for a long time, exhibiting a broad spectrum of activity against gram-positive and negative bacteria, as well as fungi. Although we would prefer a subgingival effect, the oral bacteria load reduction makes it worthwhile. The way that the essential oils are packaged into Listerine requires that it contain alcohol in order for them to work. You may have heard talk about the alcohol leading to cancer or increasing xerostomia, but those rumors have been proven not to be true. The effectiveness may not be as good as CHX but being OTC and less expensive, it will be a choice for some patients.

Cetylpyridinium chloride, which is found in Crest Pro-Health and Colgate Total, is a quaternary compound who's positive charge facilitates binding to negatively charged bacterial surfaces. This has resulted in plaque scores going down but not much of a decrease in gingival bleeding. Most oral rinses fail in their ability to attack biofilm. Free-floating bacteria are easy to kill but in their gooey matrix, they become much more difficult to kill.

Our most effective biofilm disruptors seem to be our oral rinses that contain chlorine dioxide (Oracare,

Closys). Chlorine dioxide is a powerful oxidizing agent that has been shown to penetrate the biofilm and kill off pathogenic bacteria. Additionally, the advantage of using rinses with chlorine dioxide is that they do not cause staining or altered taste and they can be used long term. Oracare is a two-part rinse that needs to be mixed, which results in a decrease in compliance. Most patients do better with Closys. It's a single bottle, it's available over the counter and patients seem to love it. For my patients, I really like Closys.

I've noticed that patients like the idea of mouthrinses doing some sort of "magic." They like easy. Their motivation and perception of the value of oral health will increase when they feel that clean, just rinsed feeling. But if it tastes bad, if it burns or if it stains, their enthusiasm will decrease and the mouthwash will be relegated to the medicine cabinet forever.

There are so many oral rinses available out there, so see what works for your patients. Experiment with different products. What works is what they should use. They almost all will have benefits and if you see good results with one particular product and the patient is happy and compliant, great!

Try to warn your patients about the possibility of staining with many of these oral rinses. But, of course, the upside of staining is that it motivates the patient to come back in for their recare appointment :)

Probiotics

In his book *Prolongation of Life* (1907), Nobel Prize winner Ellie Metchnikoff introduced the concept of probiotics. He is the first to have described the beneficial effects of bacteria, which, since Pasteur, were undeniably linked to diseases. Metchnikoff is known as the father of the probiotic concept. Probiotics are live microorganisms which, when administered in adequate amounts, confer a health benefit to the host. In ecology, this is called commensalism, which refers to a relationship between two organisms where one organism benefits from the other without affecting it. The word probiotic means "for life" as opposed to antibiotic which means "against life."

Probiotics are typically associated with the gastrointestinal tract. Our experience in dentistry has most commonly been to recommend eating yogurt (fermented dairy) to help ward off diarrhea while taking antibiotics. Besides balancing our intestinal flora, what could be the benefit of controlling the flora in our mouth? A study of an oral probiotic made by GUM (now BioGaia) called PerioBalance showed great potential for its use in helping to maintain optimal oral health. The study followed participants who received a prophylaxis, including scaling and root planing when necessary, and used one PerioBalance lozenge daily. After 60 days, there was a 43% improvement in their periodontal classification score, a 49% reduction in oral bacteria, and a 47% reduction in plaque accumulation. It seems like we are always fighting compliance and I get excited when I see products that are easy to use and pleasant. Let's face it, besides a few of our superstar patients, few people find flossing pleasant. A once a day minty lozenge, that's easy.

Exactly how probiotics work in the oral cavity is still being researched. Studies suggest that periodontal diseases may be impacted by probiotics through the reduction of the body's inflammatory response. One study found a significantly lower amount of elastase activity and lower production of matrix metalloproteinase-3 (the agent involved in the inflammatory response). Another study used two strains of L. reuteri and found a reduction in both bleeding on probing and the amount of cytokines present in the gingival crevicular fluid. This is evidence of a reduction of the body's inflammatory response, which in turn may reduce oral disease.

Probiotics are live organisms and they come in a great variety of strains. Research is required to determine which strains work in the treatment of particular health problems. The probiotic strain Lactobacillus reuteri Prodentis is a patented probiotic bacteria that is contained in BioGaia. There is quite a bit of research showing the health benefits in several areas with this probiotic. It is a naturally occurring bacterium found in human bodies, so it is a safe, natural, and side-effect-free option.

Halitosis research has shown a reduction in sulfur production among subjects using probiotic mouth rinses, lozenges, and chewing gums. Sulfur production contributes to halitosis, and when the probiotic S. salivarius K12 was used, a reduction occurred. A similar study was performed using a strain of L. salivarius. They found a noticeable decrease in halitosis after two and four weeks of consumption.

ProBioraPro from ProBiora Health contains Streptococcus oralis, Streptococcus uberis, and Streptococcus rattus. These strains come originally from the oral flora. These three strains have been shown to be effective in reducing periodontitis as well as caries. The magic of this probiotic is that these strains of Strep don't produce lactic acid which cause cavities but instead produce hydrogen peroxide that kills periodontal pathogens.

Does your dog have bad breath? They make ProBioraPet just for him. Probiotics, sprinkled over Fido's food, will decrease doggy breath noticeably.

Probiotics can play a crucial role in halting, altering, or delaying periodontal diseases if we let them. It poses great potential in the arena of periodontics in terms of plaque modification, halitosis management, altering anaerobic bacteria colonization, improvement of pocket depth, and clinical attachment loss. Let's not keep this helper away from our patients. They can be found over the counter or online and are easy to use. Because probiotics contain live microorganisms and antibiotics are designed to kill certain bacteria, probiotics should be taken no sooner than two hours following administration of the antibiotic.

Be patient, they will need to be taken for a couple of weeks before any significant changes are noticed. This microscopic army is ready to help your patients fight off the bad guys. Try it and see how they work for your patients.

Salivary Diagnostics

Spit, is it more than just something to drool down our face or suck up with our saliva ejector? The future of medical diagnostics is right in front of our nose (or more accurately), right below our nose. It is saliva. Most compounds found in blood are also found in saliva because saliva is the result of specialized cells taking up water, salts and macromolecules from the blood, mixing them with a cocktail of saliva-specific proteins and flowing out of our parotid, submandibular, and sublingual salivary glands. Some substances may also reach saliva by passing from blood through the spaces between the cells. This means that our saliva provides all of the information necessary for detecting a range of natural and artificial substances, such as proteins, electrolytes, hormones, antibodies, DNA/RNA, therapeutic medications, and recreational drugs. This can indicate the health of the immune system, nutritional defects, and metabolic states, neurological conditions, as well as emotional and hormonal status.

So, you might be wondering why you have been having your blood drawn and your urine collected. These tests have been used routinely as a medical screening and diagnostic tool for a good reason: molecular diagnoses are based on blood samples that contain high concentrations of the molecules of interest. But technology has given us newer, more sensitive tests, enabling the detection of very small amounts of these substances which makes salivary diagnostics a current reality. Ready access to saliva is helpful for one-time sample collection, and an even greater benefit when multiple or serial sampling is required, such as for the ongoing, real-time assessment of health and disease status.

In our office, we can have a patient swish with a saline solution and spit it into a tube. We send it off and within a few days, we get the results. For periodontal disease, we test for the levels of pathogenic bacteria. We get a report back that shows us which bacteria are present and whether they are over the threshold levels that put a patient at risk for periodontal disease. With this, we can create an individualized plan to lower the levels of the different strains of bacteria, whether it is with systemic antibiotics, clinical treatment, and/or home care. We can assess our progress by retesting 6-8 weeks later. Don't be surprised when you see the test for one person comes back almost identical to their partner's. We constantly reinfect those that we are affectionate towards, creating very similar bacterial profiles.

Some of the salivary tests that are available to be performed in a dental office are the detection of pathogenic bacteria, periodontal disease susceptibility through genetic markers, human papillomavirus (HPV)/

oral cancer, herpes simplex virus (HSV), creatinine reactive protein (CRP) and human immunodeficiency virus (HIV). Currently, the process does require sending the specimens to a laboratory for processing, but the future is being developed right now at UCLA where they are creating in-office, real-time saliva testing. Can you imagine that instead of relying on bleeding on probing and bone loss to determine the state of disease you could have a patient give a saliva sample and all of the earliest markers are quantified right there before our eyes? Wow!

Salivary diagnostics will dramatically change the clinical practice of dentistry because, as you know, most of our patients see us more often than their physician, and who other than dental professionals has such a keen focus on prevention? But first, there will be challenges: the education of the dental profession regarding the conditions for which the tests are designed, reimbursement issues and practice implications. Will dental offices embrace a broader base of medical diagnostics, such as screening for breast cancer, chronic disease or drug use, rather than a focus on tests for oral conditions like dental caries and periodontal disease? I think they will. Someday, taking a saliva sampling in a dental clinic will become as routine as obtaining a urine or blood sample at a physician's office.

Most importantly, the appeal of salivary diagnostics is to detect disease at the earliest stage. Honestly, as our insurance "partners" would like us to do, treating periodontal disease after radiographic bone loss is visualized is just too darn late. Biomarkers of biofilm, inflammation, collagen breakdown and bone remodeling are all present, right there in the spit! And if we detect breast cancer at its earliest stage of development, you, the superstar, may have saved another life.

Floss Alternatives

By a show of hands, how many of you have ever had a patient tell you to never to use the f word (floss) around them again, or been told that "I do floss, every day" (really?), or by rote, have told a patient "you need to floss more" (knowing good and well that there's no way they're going to do that), or decided not to mention floss to a patient because you know they just aren't listening? I had a patient that said, "Every time I drive past your office I feel guilty about not flossing"(not that it has affected his sporadic flossing habit). Have you ever run into a patient at the supermarket and had them be embarrassed about their oral hygiene right there in the middle of the dog food aisle when they saw you ("Oh I need to floss more"). The guilt is at an all-time high. A recent study found that 27% of patients lie to us about their flossing habits! Yet, we keep banging our heads against the wall.

One of my first patients ever in dental school was Mr. Stuhley. An older guy, retired, big beer belly, bald head, big smile, very happy all the time, just a great guy, but boy were his gums a mess. The kind of gums you only see in school. He professed his love for flossing and recited like a schoolboy that he brushed twice a day for two minutes and flossed every night. Ok, I'm thinking, then there is obviously a technique problem. "Mr. Stuhley, could you show me exactly how you floss?" I handed him the floss and within thirty seconds he had it wrapped around his fingers, his elbows, his neck, and his right ear. I jumped in to stop him since I was still shaky on my CPR skills. Could he, Mr. Stuhley, have been lying to me?

Since only 10-15% of the American population floss (which is probably the percentage of hygienists in America :)), we have to look at alternatives to flossing. Studies do support this move away from flossing. I'm not looking to convert people who already floss to something else, but what should we offer the other 85%?

How about interdental cleaning devices like wooden tips, interproximal brushes, and rubber tip stimulators? These have been shown to be quite effective. Those that use these seem to be pretty committed to oral hygiene, the sort of person that would floss if they could, if it wasn't so hard, if it wasn't so complicated. Yes, flossing is way more complicated than we think. You have to step beyond your gift of adept hand skills and realize that the average person is a klutz. Adapting the floss around the mesial of the distal tooth and the distal of the mesial tooth is more difficult for our patients than we can ever imagine. Trying to remember that the bridge can't be flossed between the abutment and the pontic no matter how hard they try to push through seems like it should be pretty straight forward. Remembering that the floss they bought at the dollar store isn't really that good but maybe it is better than the kite string they just tried to use is a start. Like with flossing, it is wise to watch how the patient handles whatever it is that they like to use and make sure that their technique is effective.

Can anyone tell me why we are so hung up on floss? Is it the "gold standard" of home care? There have been serious concerns with flossing, namely, hardly anyone (hygienists excluded) do it correctly, maybe no one. Secondly, we are passing microbes from one site to the next. Thirdly, anatomical concavities like the interproximals of maxillary bicuspids and molars are completely missed. Fourthly, how much gingival stimulation are we getting, especially compared to an oral irrigator like a Waterpik Water Flosser®, proxy brush or Go-Between? And finally, floss doesn't wash out, lavage, the site. Oral irrigators have a similar benefit of that of an ultrasonic scaler; flushing out pathogens. We are seeing the crown passed to oral irrigators.

Yes, I love oral irrigators. They are easy to use, effective and they feel good to use. So why are so many of them bought and left under the sink or unused on the countertop? A few reasons come to mind.

The number one complaint is about them being messy (water spots on the bathroom mirror in some households can start a huge fight). This is usually only a problem as a person is starting to learn how to use it. Time and experience will make that complaint disappear along with gingival bleeding. But if a person just can't master splatter-less oral irrigator usage, Waterpik makes a travel one that works well if you want to multitask during your daily shower. This will allow freedom from unsightly water drops on the mirror!

Another reason is that it does take some effort and like flossing or any home care, it is our responsibility to educate our patients about the importance of daily irrigation. Don't just say you have to do this or your teeth could fall out, come up with your own visual. For example, "Imagine, if you will, what will happen tonight if you don't remove this bacteria that I am showing you here in the mirror. They will gang up, marinate and then burrow into your gums releasing sulfur gas which will not only make your breath stink tomorrow but will make your gums dissolve."

Lastly, oral irrigator use correlates with the hygienist's belief in them. Studies show that Waterpik Water Flosser® is 29% better than floss for overall plaque removal and 51% more effective than floss for reducing gingivitis. The studies have been around since 2009, so what's the hold-up? These statistics compare Water Flossers to flossing, but we need to compare Water Flossers to not flossing. Water Flossers are easier to use, so we have a much better chance of getting our patients to use a Water Flosser rather than traditional flossing. Patients will say they like it, and they really feel the difference. Try it for yourself and you will be a believer. Watch your patients that are using one and see the results with your own eyes. It is astounding!

There are other oral irrigators on the market. Sonicare Air Flosser is quite popular, but, the Waterpik Water Flosser has been shown to be 30% more effective than it. Though, if a person likes it, is using it, and doesn't want to change, it is still way more effective than doing nothing. Hydro Floss is very similar to the Water Flosser® but it adds a magnet to magnetize the water. Just as magnets have been shown to reduce calcium and lime deposits in plumbing, research has shown that it can reduce supragingival plaque and calculus by 44%.

Let's keep our eyes open for new products, products that our patients will use. It will feel uncomfortable at first, but you really can tell your patient that they don't have to floss. They will welcome the relief from the f word and embrace the alternatives. Patients love it when I tell them that they don't need to floss and that they don't need to feel guilty about it either. All they have to do is pick up an oral irrigator like a Water Flosser or Hydro Floss. Done.

How many patients don't come back because they don't want to be yelled at and beaten up for not flossing?

Powered Toothbrushes

I can't think of another product that my patients love as much as their powered toothbrushes. I don't know what it is. It is probably the feeling that they get, the "just had my teeth cleaned" feeling, or it could be the encouragement we give them when we see the improvement in their oral health. For me, I like it for the efficiency. Love the bass technique but I sure can't get my manual toothbrush to oscillate, rotate and pulse at the rate of these fine electric ones. For me, I like the mindlessness of the timer telling me when to switch to a different area, allowing me to multitask in the morning, brushing my teeth as I try to find matching socks. I'll even use it in the shower, giving me an excuse to stay in the warm shower longer. I guess that would count for leaving the water running when you brush, whoops. Very few people won't appreciate a good mechanical brushing.

All of the common misconceptions of powered toothbrushes have been disproven. No, a manual one can't keep up with a powered toothbrush in removing plaque. No, powered toothbrushes are not more abrasive, causing more recession. No, they don't cause more toothbrushing injuries. But, yes, they are great for people with disabilities, dexterity problems and for children. Compliance is very good, and people are brushing longer.

So what could be the controversy? I hear dental professionals touting one brush over the other. Maybe one is slightly better than the other, but does it matter? I don't see it. They are all quite effective. The more advanced (expensive) brushes do perform a bit better than the cheaper ones but they all beat a manual brush. I think that it is more important that a person uses one that they like. As an office, I like to have everyone recommending the same toothbrushes so that it minimizes the consumer confusion and gives a stronger recommendation than, "Just get any one of those electric brushes." I'd rather hear, "Today, on your way home from this appointment, do yourself and your health a favor and invest in a (fill in the blank) toothbrush, it will change your life, it will save your life, and the next time that you're in, I'll be able to pat you on the back for the improvement in your health."

Local and Systemic Antibiotics

Periodontitis, the most common chronic inflammatory condition known to mankind, is a disease that results in the destruction of tooth-supporting tissues. This destruction comes from the body's inflammatory response to the periodontal pathogens. Since the chain of events goes from the formation of a bacterial biofilm on the tooth surface below the gingival margin to our body's inflammatory response (host response), to the destruction of the collagen making up the periodontal ligament and other periodontal tissues, we can attack the problem in two different ways. One way is to decrease the pathogenic bacteria and the other is to decrease our host response (decrease our inflammatory response). Decreasing our inflammatory response is called host modulation therapy (HMT).

Antibiotic therapy success has commonly been attributed to its bactericidal properties, but research has been shown that tetracyclines have an additional property. The tetracyclines also exhibit the ability to disrupt the inflammatory response by down-regulating one of the enzymes that is responsible for causing tissue destruction. This makes the tetracyclines not only an antimicrobial but also an anti-inflammatory. This is why they have been so successful in treating chronic periodontitis in the past. But, keeping a patient on an antibiotic for extended lengths of time can lead to diminishing returns, as bacterial resistance grows.

This has led to the development of Periostat, a subantimicrobial dose of doxycycline (SDD). The idea is to use a tetracycline in the form of doxycycline, in a dose that won't affect the bacteria, but still has the ability to work as an anti-inflammatory, reducing the patient's excessive inflammatory response to the bacterial exposure. So, the two-pronged approach is to reduce the bacterial load by scaling and root planing and then using 20 mg of doxycycline twice a day for 3-24 months. Modern thinking suggests that successful, long term management of chronic periodontitis should combine both local mechanical and subantimicrobial strategies.

Another anti-inflammatory antibiotic is Azithromycin (Zithromax). In medicine, it has been used extensively for the treatment of a wide range of infections such as upper respiratory tract infections and middle ear infections. It is also effective against the most common periodontal pathogens. Azithromycin is in the class of antibiotics known as macrolides, which because of its ability to reduce inflammation, is used to treat diseases not associated with bacteria, such as severe asthma, chronic obstructive pulmonary diseases and, more recently, cystic fibrosis. Studies show favorable results for the use of a single course (three tablets) of azithromycin in the treatment of advanced periodontal diseases. Azithromycin could have a triple role in the treatment and resolution of periodontal diseases: suppressing pathogenic bacteria, anti-inflammatory activity and healing through persistence at low levels in macrophages and fibroblasts in periodontal tissues. These properties also make it very beneficial in cases of drug-induced gingival enlargement.

There have been several locally applied subgingival antimicrobials that have made their way to the market. A resorbable gelatin matrix containing chlorhexidine gluconate called PerioChip has been around for a while with some good results. It releases CHX for 7-10 days and has been shown to improve pocket depths and bleeding for over nine months. Subgingival doxycycline (Atridox) and subgingval minocycline (Arestin) have seen similar positive results including reduction of bleeding points, increase in clinical attachment level and probing depths. These subgingival antimicrobials should always be used as adjuncts to scaling and root planing. This will ensure that there will be a reduction in bacteria as well as in the body's inflammatory response.

We know that some people are more susceptible to periodontal disease. This is due to an environmental or genetic predisposition that provokes the body to have an excessive response to the pathogenic insult. The idea of modulating the host response is heating up with research hoping to not just help with periodontal disease, but also other inflammatory diseases like rheumatoid arthritis and inflammatory bowel disease. More products are on the way, so keep an eye out for the exciting new advances in host modulation therapy and be the first one in your town to understand and use these innovative treatments.

Healthy Gums Don't Bleed

Does it make sense that gums should bleed? Bleeding tells us that there has been a breakdown in the epithelial lining in our periodontal pockets. This can now allow those periodontal pathogens to invade the sulcular tissue, and jump into our vascular system to be carried away to other sites and wreak havoc in ways we just couldn't have imagined in the past.

When we do our charting and we see that we have gotten a reduction in the number of bleeding sites, in the past we felt good. Yes, we have decreased the systemic inflammation and consequentially their systemic risk of disease, but how about now? Are we good with that? Is it ok that we have any bleeding? We have seen how one site can infect another site, so having one or two areas pumping out potentially fatal bacterial pathogens into our system should alarm us.

Take a stand, don't accept any amount of bleeding. But also, don't worry. If you're thinking, I know, but I have these patients that no matter what I do they are still going to be a mess, they are going to bleed. We have a plan. Use these products and procedures to help you with your fight. And develop the necessary communication skills so that you can motivate your patients to not only understand what optimal oral health looks like but to want it. Your patients will develop a new appreciation for what you do and for what they do at home.

If they won't do more, then we may have to be more creative. Rethink what we do. There is some thought that a monthly coronal polishing may have a positive outcome in the reduction of inflammation and the progression of periodontal disease. Can you think of a patient that you would like to try this on? Try it out, take notes and see what results you get. Let's be creative. Let's find out what a patient can do, make them feel good about coming in for their appointment and then do what we can do: educate, motivate and inspire, all without guilt. But we need to keep the truth in mind, we need to take a stand…

Healthy Gums Don't Bleed!

Section Seven
FOR WHAT YOU ARE WORTH

by Coach Steve

Every time you state what you want or believe, you're the first to hear it. It's a message to both you and others about what you think is possible. Don't put a ceiling on yourself.

– Oprah Winfrey

Your Vision of a Healthier World

The greatest gift of having a vision to follow is the confidence it gives you. You know that it's the right thing to do because it comes from who you are. So this fuel for your journey will take you to heights that others, who are sitting on their hands, will only be able to wonder about. At the same time, you will still be asking yourself, "What is my lifetime body of work? What am I the proudest of? Can I do more? Do I have more to share?" I know you do.

The journey is long, and sometimes you may need to draw upon this confidence to overcome occasional doubts and insecurities. Maybe it feels weird to be leading instead of following. That's OK. You can do it. Your vision is giving you a full tank. Your vision is that important. It is worth fighting for. It is that strong. Nothing, including self-doubt, insecurity, discomfort, or burn out, is a match for your vision. Your important, meaningful vision will squash any negativity that gets in its way.

Did you ever have a coach who got the very best out of you? Did that coach YELL, "End strong!?" Did that coach believe in you? Your vision is that coach, and it needs you. The movement needs you. Don't finish weak or slow. Let's get this thing done. It is too important to stop now. We need to leave this world a better place. We can do it. We got this.

Believe In Yourself

Believe in yourself! Let's start with something fun. Body language. Everyone loves body language and nonverbal communication. Do you keep your chin raised while talking? Do you make yourself big while making a point? Do you stand tall and wide when speaking? Do you make eye contact? Interestingly, that's what you are supposed to do when you are in the wild. If you lay down in a ball in the wild, you will become lunch. If you are not familiar with power posing or Dr. Amy Cuddy, please find her TED Talk on YouTube. It's definitely worth the twenty minutes.

Confidence comes from believing in yourself, your industry, and the science. Confidence is situational. Confidence becomes influential when you believe. Do you believe? How much bleeding on probing is acceptable? You know this... Do you believe it? I don't want to sound dated, but Stuart Smalley said, "I am good enough, I am smart enough, and doggone it, people like me." That was his mantra for success. I believe in you.

Belief comes from that deep place inside you where you just know... Not the same as faith exactly. What would you give someone who gives you hope? Hope to be better. Hope that the answer is out there. That oral health and overall health are connected. That everything can be better. That your immune system can be stronger.

That you can effect simple things like the common cold in a positive way. The chance of contracting a life-threatening disease is less. Why don't you believe? I believe in you.

When you believe it, you will see it! When you believe something is impossible, your mind goes to work to prove why it is impossible. But, when you believe, really believe something can be done, your mind helps you find ways to do it.

Believing something can be done paves the way for creative solutions. To help yourself develop creative power, eliminate the word "impossible" from your vocabulary. "Impossible," "never," "can't," "not in a million years," "did that and it didn't work," these are all failure words. Those thoughts set off a chain reaction, which works to prove that it is impossible.

Traditional thinking will kill today's dental industry. If dentistry is to survive and improve patients' health, then creative leaders, dentists, hygienists, and teams must change. Did you know that nothing grows in ice? If we let tradition "freeze" our minds, new ideas can't sprout. Propose one of the ideas below to someone in the dental industry and watch their reaction:

- You must cut your overhead by 40% today.
- Staff the office from 7 a.m. until 7 p.m.
- Case acceptance is 100%, no exceptions.

- All Americans will seek dental care this year.

Whether or not these statements are practical, what's important is how a person handles these propositions. If they laugh at the idea without giving it a second thought (and probably 95% will laugh at you), chances are they suffer from tradition paralysis. The one in twenty who says, "I'm open to that," "That's an interesting idea," or, "Tell me more about it" has a mind open to creativity.

Traditional thinking is Enemy Number One for the dental team interested in future success. Traditional thinking "freezes" your mind, blocks your progress, and prevents you from developing creative power. Here are three ways to fight it:

1. Become receptive to ideas. Welcome new ideas and concepts. Say, "I'm open to that." Success has very little to do with how smart you are. "We may not be the smartest dental team, but we listen and soak up all the great ideas out there."
2. Be an experimental team. Expose yourself to new learning. Try new ideas.
3. Be progressive, not regressive. Don't say, "That's the way we did it at my old office. We ought to do it that way here." Ask yourself, "How can we do it better than before?"

Questions we should continue to ask ourselves and find answers for:

- How can I make a difference today?
- What can I do today to encourage my team?
- What special favor can I do for one of my patients today?
- How can I change a life today?
- How can I be that "change agent" today?
- What is great about our team?
- What isn't great yet?
- What are the most exciting things going on at work?
- How can we increase profit pay this month and have fun doing it?
- How can the team support our cause for healthy lives?

Home

Earlier I said, find your home. Your home is where you are appreciated. Home is where you have an owner who pays you what you're worth. Home is where you are loved, empowered, and asked to lead. Your home should feel right. Your home should be your happy place. Your home is where you are most confident. Home is where you are supported even when you are wrong. Home can be where you are. Home is not always elsewhere. The old saying, "The grass is always greener on the other side," is not necessarily true. Grass is greener wherever you water and fertilize it. Water and fertilize yourself and your team. Do everything in your power to make your current place your home. If you are not in that place of joy and happiness, then leave. It is better to leave than stay. It takes courage to leave. Please leave… You are not serving yourself, your team, or your patients. You know it is true. Have the courage to leave.

How to get that superstar job… Don't work for money, work for knowledge. Don't make money the reason to NOT get your dream job. Come into the opportunity with the right attitude. Take responsibility to earn your place and income. Be humble but confident. They want you, and they need you. When you introduce yourself to that new dentist, don't ask for an interview. Dentists hate the pressure of the interview. Ask for an introduction, meet and greet, or just a conversation of possibility. Attitude determines altitude. Don't expect much from your first visit. Yes, stop by personally. Yes, "secret shop" all of the dental offices in your area prior to stopping by. It still amazes me how much I learn from one phone call. The entire culture comes through the phone. Listen for the signs of a happy, progressive team.

After you call every office, drop in to hand-deliver your letter of introduction. Letter of introduction, not resume or CV. The introduction letter should be a request to meet the Dr only. You have heard great things from others in the area and would like to introduce yourself. The letter should include a picture. Not a picture of you in scrubs but a picture of you doing what you love: tennis, golf, with your family, kids, dogs. Out of respect, most dentists will meet you. You need to have that attitude of thank you and do you have any advice for me? Both where to go, and where not to go. Who is progressive in the market, and who is old school. Who is marketing, and who is staying pat… Knowledge is power. Get to know your market. The more meet and greets you get, the better the chance of finding your home. If the meet and greet goes well, make sure to get their opinion on pay. Ask, "I have heard a range of pay in the area of _____ to _____. Is that what you would consider fair?" Ask about benefits as well. Tell them you want to be super fair so you can get a chance to earn your pay. You want to give back, not take away…

Always have a goal at your meet and greet. Can you ask for over the shoulder time in office? Can you attend a team meeting? Can you attend a huddle meeting? Can you fill in for vacation or sick days? Ask for a favor when you leave. Ask for help. Ask the doctor and team to keep their eyes open to your new awesome home. Above all, have fun along the journey of finding your new home. Smile and laugh when appropriate. Share your knowledge only when asked.

When you get your interview make sure to ask the owner questions. They will respect you more if you know what to ask. Here are some simple sample questions you should ask:

Who has influenced your model of practicing dentistry?

I love this question… Broad and open-ended. Listen to the answer. Do they start with clinical?, marketing?, or practice management? Let them speak. Ask them their "story." Listen, listen, listen.

What dental work do you refer out?

I have found this to be the easiest way to determine a practice's clinical care and philosophy. Do they keep it all? What are they skilled and confident in doing? What have they continued to study and learn?

What are your thoughts about periodontal disease?

Similar to yours?

How active is your perio program?

Make sure to follow up with number of quads 4341 they do, and how many patients are in perio maintenance 4910.

Do you pre-appoint?

Does your hygienist do it in the back, or does front office do it? Do you know your percentage of patients that pre-appointed? It takes 1 hour to track down a patient and schedule them if they don't leave with an appointment. Share your knowledge. They will love you for it! If not, make sure you tell them you want to. The more you do the more efficient the team is.

What is your protocol on digital photography?

Make sure they know YOU know how critical photos are and how committed you are to getting a full series of photos on all patients.

What do you love doing as a dentist?

Great question here. By listening to what they love you learn what they don't love. Make sure to communicate your skills in the areas they don't like.

Have you had or currently have a coach?

If they have never had one your job may be difficult. The very best in everything have multiple coaches. The do-it-yourself dentists will be hard to influence. What kind of coaching? Clinical? Practice management? Marketing? Was it positive or negative?

Where do you see yourself five years from now?

If they don't know you can't help them get there... It's no fun to repeat the same day over and over again like Groundhog Day!

What is your vision of dentistry?

Occasionally I meet that superstar dentist who gets it. They know what is coming. They know the influence of corporate dentistry. They know the marketing game. They know how valuable the team is. They are always looking for YOU! Even if they don't have a spot for you. This may be your home...

What is your mission, vision, and goals for this year?

Does it excite you?

What do you know about the oral-systemic health

link?

Possible deal breaker?

Who you are looking for is looking for you! You will find that home. You will be in that happy place. We got this. We can make this happen. Say YES slowly when looking. Leave quickly when you are not in your correct home.

Getting Paid What You're Worth

What are you worth? I taught my children to have a "pat" answer to this one. "I am WORTH MILLIONS. I just haven't talked anyone into paying me that yet!" Let me start by declaring that I believe you are under-loved and underpaid. Seriously, I do believe that. I think you hold all the cards. They're in your passion and your ability to get patients to believe you, like you, and trust you (BLT). I also believe that some of you have a harder time finding jobs than others. Some of you get paid more than others, although most of you are in that average range. The best of you can ask the owner to sign your check, and you put the amount in.

How do you negotiate your worth? What is your value? What is the fair market value (FMV plus Profit Pay) in your market? Fair market value is not determined by the doctor, by the coach, or by you. FMV is determined by what the market will pay. If you take ten of your friends and average the high and the low, that is FMV. Why get paid high fair market value? Why settle for what the market pays? Why NOT get paid like a Superstar!?

So how can you break the mold? Throw away the standard FMV plus Profit Pay. Make a difference and prove it! The proof is in the pudding. You learn how to create value and how to become indispensable to your practice. Become a Superstar Hygienist and learn to get paid for it. When hygienists base value and pay on what they produce as a provider in the hygiene department, I laugh. That is not your value. The company will never get rich on $1,500/days or even $2,500/days. That is not your true value. That is not what you should attach your pay to. How do YOU have a $5,000 day? How about a $50,000/day? You have them all the time. Your value is getting patients to believe you, like you, and trust you (BLT). When patients believe you, like you, and trust you, they will do whatever you ask of them. More work is diagnosed out of your treatment room than you realize. More importantly, you forever change lives.

It is shortsighted to attach your pay to dollars produced by you. That is not where dentists make money. They earn income directly from total work done. 60%-75% comes from operative dentistry. Income is not your only value. You need to understand wealth. Wealth is created when the owner sells the practice. Depending on how he sells the practice, it can be worth 3.2 to 11 times the earnings. Wow! 100% of the value of dental offices is based on the quality of active patients, the ability to transfer the relationships, and net income. The quality relationship happens to be YOU. Quality relationships are the patients who pre-appoint and come back to see YOU or one of your team members. All of my practices understand Wealth! They don't just work for income. They work for Wealth.

Wealth is created by the number of patients seen in hygiene per month. Track it. Grow it! It's not uncommon for practices to grow from 250 patients seen in hygiene to 500 patients seen. It's fun for me to watch practices grow and grow. At 200 patients seen, the average dentists can't provide care to establish the availability and access that consumers want. I recommend adding an associate at 200 hygiene patients and 25 new patients per month. So many dentists don't run their practice to accommodate growth. You will make sure the practice stays ahead of growth. Growth is how we create income and wealth. Persuade your dentist to allow you to run your department. That includes growth. That includes income and wealth. If you don't have the skills to do this, then get them. This is your house. This is your business. Treat your department like that and get paid like a superstar.

Negotiating is critical to your success and happiness. I want to list several things that you can do to help yourself. What is the fair market value in your market? Don't ask your professor at your school (whatever he tells you is probably wrong). Ask your friends. Make a diligent effort to find out. Then find out what the doctor knows, where he/she got his information and when he/she got it. You need to know what he/she knows. My advice is to always understand that the doctor does not know you, and initially the risk is with the office.

What if you asked for $30/hour or even $25/hour for the first month (way UNDER value) to show your worth.

It is interesting to me that you would take a job without interviewing the team and doctor. Forget that at the end of 30 days you may not want to stay. It makes so much sense to negotiate your value after you show your skills and see if they are worthy of you! I would ask for below ridiculous pay so you can get that review in 30 days. Make sure your intentions are clear. If you want $50-$60 (yes superstars are worth that) make sure they know the range you are looking for. Eliminate money as the reason to not hire you, then prove your worth.

Profit pay is an interesting question and different in all practices. Typically profit pay is a team distribution for going above the bare minimum. Most dentists call this a bonus. I don't like the bonus concept because it perpetuates entitlement by the team. When a formula is used it is not based on profit but production or collections. We want to be paid profit. Always use the word profit when speaking to the owner. Do not go All-In on a team bonus. The team eventually will hold you back. I want my offices to pay half of the total available dollars as team profit pay and the other half individually to the superstars. As an example of profit pay… Varnish costs $3-$5, and we can charge $20-$40. Ask your dentist to pay you $5 per paid application. Pretty easy for an owner to say yes to this. Good for the patient. Good for the owner. Good for the hygienist.

"Keep what you kill" is an expression used to communicate pay based on results. My clients will never pay 50%, 40% or even 30% of your adjusted production. If you can negotiate "keep what you kill," go for it. Get paid in direct proportion to your dollars generated. If money is your goal, this may be the best way to get paid. Unlimited upside and unlimited downside. Take responsibility for your results. Personally, I don't think it's the right method: it is shortsighted and hurts the team, owner, and patients. It creates too many leadership and management issues. It creates a scarcity mentality. We want an abundance mentality. It is selfish and not fulfilling to work for just the money. Most hygienists work to serve others, serving them as a friend, counselor, and health care provider. Most of you work for the love of the game. To make a difference. To change lives and to save lives. If that is you, then consider developing value for what you do for the practice. Dentists love it when you get a patient excited about their restorative or cosmetic treatment needs while in your chair. When you close an Invisalign case, cosmetic case, or implant case, your value grows exponentially.

What percentage of patients pre-appoint out of your room? Do you take personal responsibility to make this happen in your room? You should if you want to maximize praise and pay. Show your worth and value to the owner. Remember, the quality of your relationships gives the dental practice its value. That is YOUR relationship with your patients. Track the percentage pre-appointed. It better be 95%+. If not, get training to get it there. Don't rely on your team to do this. Your patients will be more committed to you or another hygiene team member. Remember it is a family practice. You don't own the patients. You want access and availability to be the culture. Your job is to make everyone else look awesome. When you pre-appoint make sure the patient schedule comes first. Pre-appoint into someone else's day. Wow, that is a superstar hygienist.

Resentful dentists are not what you want. Life is too short to have a dentist resent what he pays you. Even the dentists I work with need to be reminded of who the superstars are and why. Knowing your value is critical. I hope this book gives you some sense of how we value YOU! If asked, I answer quickly that your value is based on three things: trust and rapport with your patients (BLT), asking comprehensive questions (case acceptance), and fulfilling on hygiene treatment needed.

When asked for the long version, this is the answer:

- Know your numbers and review end of day sheets (patients pre-appointed, seen, dollars, pictures, handoffs, work diagnosed, accepted).
- Ask comprehensive questions of patient health (sleep apnea, risk factors, Invisalign, cosmetic, restorative, perio, overall health) and "transfer of power" to the Doctor.
- Use the Total Care Interview process to "transfer power," educate, and handoff patients

throughout the team.
- Be happy, smile, and maintain that superstar attitude toward your team, doctor, and patients.
- Attend daily huddle meetings prepared with information specific to yesterday (big rocks) and today.
- Keep patients active and committed to pre-appointing and office confirmation protocols.
- Have daily huddle meetings with a Hygiene Coordinator (if you have never worked with one, come to one of our programs).
- Help fill cancellations and no shows (coordinate with Hygiene Coordinator).
- Teach patients ideal home care.
- BLT- Believability, Likability, and Trust!
- Promote all marketing efforts to grow the practice (reviews, video testimonials, asking for referrals, raffles, family members past due).
- Communicate effectively with all team members.
- Hold monthly meetings with your Hygiene Coordinator to review department effectiveness and goals.
- Support the Hygiene Coordinator efforts to pre-appoint ALL patients (ER, patients seen by Dr).
- Take patients' photos/x-rays and show educational videos/materials as needed and have them ready for the doctor to review.

- Keep the treatment room clean and set up for each procedure.
- Keep instruments sharp, clean, and sterile.
- Inform Clinical Assistant of needed equipment and supplies to order.
- Be motivated and show your team how a superstar acts.
- The most critical thing to remember is to BELIEVE! Believe in yourself. Believe in Science. Believe in living a quality, healthy, happy life.

Dentists don't know what they don't know. It is your job to tell them. It is your job to make your value to the business indispensable. You are worth millions! Let's make sure your dentist knows that…

Learn more becoming the best, becoming a Hygiene Superstar.
HygieneSuperstar.com/superstar

Hygiene Superstar

Section Eight
FOR YOUR DENTIST
by Dr. Mike

If you have knowledge, let others light their candles in it.

– **Margaret Fuller**

How fortunate it is to have a team member who cares so much about your patients and your practice. She/he is one of the special hygienists interested in improving the lives of your patients by joining a movement called Complete Health Dentistry. Maybe you've heard of it. It stems from the relatively young organization the American Academy for Oral Systemic Health (AAOSH). It is a movement of dental professionals who are dedicated to taking dentistry and patient health to a higher level.

Chronic disease, most of which is entirely preventable, costs our country over $1 trillion a year. Inflammation is the root cause of this, and we now have great studies that show that periodontal pathogens living in our patients' mouths exacerbate the devastation. My father had his first heart attack at the age of 48 and survived that one only because he was across the street from the UCLA medical center. He did die from a heart attack at the age of 60. No, he didn't smoke. He didn't have an unhealthy lifestyle. What he did have was a huge inflammatory burden on his body. He had rheumatoid arthritis and periodontal disease. Back then I didn't know that there was a connection between them, and truth be told, I resisted the connection for a long time, even after the floss or die movement. I knew that there was a positive correlation between heart disease and periodontal disease, but I was not convinced that reducing periodontal disease would make the heart any healthier. I am convinced now. In 2016, periodontal pathogens were proven to cause arterial disease. The mechanism of bacteria going from a periodontal pocket, through the bloodstream, and ending up in the arterial wall where it gets cholesterol to accumulate into deadly plaques is now proven and documented. In fact, a recent study showed that up to 50% of heart attacks are triggered by oral infections. People are suffering because medicine is focused so much on treatment rather than prevention.

As dentists and hygienists, we are in the perfect place to have a more positive effect on the health of our patients. Generally, our patients see us more often than they see their GP. We have a better relationship with them, and we are much more preventive minded. So many of our patients have the old school belief that heart attacks are caused by a "clog," like in a drain, when in fact the vast majority come from plaques throwing a clot that then occludes a vessel, causing either a heart attack or stroke. With more modern views of inflammation, bacterial biofilm, and treatment regimens, it is crucial that our hygiene departments evolve.

Honestly, I never thought of perio as being that sexy. It wasn't the CE class I was lining up for. I thought I was doing a fine job, doing what I'd learned back in the '80s in school (which hasn't changed much). Then I went to my first AAOSH meeting and, wow, I will never again practice the same way. I see perio in a whole new light. My patients are excited, and my team is excited, which makes me even more excited.

As well as so many of our patients, so many of our loved ones have a family history of heart disease or stroke, diabetes, or cancer. You owe it to yourself and them to make sure you are knowledgeable about this oral/systemic connection. Once you do, the idea of moving your practice towards a Complete Health Dentistry will be a natural one.

Hygienists get this stuff. They want to be Hygiene Superstars. They want the best for you, your practice, and for your patients. They can use your help by being open-minded and empowering them to help improve the scope and quality of the treatment in the hygiene department.

Although this book was written for your hygienists, I hope that you, the dentist, will find it interesting and inspiring.

No longer are we just saving teeth. We are saving lives. It feels good. It feels right.

Acknowledgements

Firstly, we would like to thank Susan Wingrove, RDH, BS for her inspiration, guidance, and encouragement. Stephanie Lodding, RDH for her energy and passion. Jan Lazarus, RDH, HC for opening up our eyes and for her bravery to talk oral/systemic way before it was cool. All the amazing minds in AAOSH for constantly pushing us forward. And, of course, the Hygiene Superstars at Camarillo Smiles for their openmindedness and commitment to the vision.

We are both very lucky to be fueled by the support of two amazing wives: Dianne Sperry and Mindy Czubiak who have been there for us for over 30 years.

Heartfelt thanks(pun intended) to Amy Doneen, DNP, ARNP and Brad Bale, MD for exposing inflammation as public enemy #1. And, for empowering and saving so many genetically condemned patients like us. We are eternally grateful to Chris Kammer, DDS and all of the founders of AAOSH for recognizing the need to blur the distinction between medicine and dentistry.

And finally, thank you to editors Sebastian Sarti and Elena Czubiak for making it seem like we know what an Oxford comma is.

About The Authors

Dr. Mike Czubiak:

Dr. Mike is a practicing general dentist in Camarillo, California. He graduated from UCLA in 1988 and started his own practice from scratch. He grew his practice by recognizing the importance of a strong preventive program and top-notch dental hygienists. His team now includes nine hygiene superstars. Dr. Czubiak has lectured extensively on technology, practice management, and leadership and has brought fresh solutions to dental teams throughout the US. He is the founder of Camarillo Smiles, the California Academy of Dental Assisting, and co-founder of Lotus-Leadership for Dentists. He can be heard on his podcasts Uncomfortable Dental Conversations with co-author Coach Steve and the Hygiene Superstar podcast with Dr. Tom Larkin.

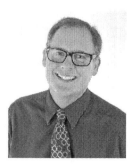

Saving teeth is good, saving lives is better.
-Dr. Mike Czubiak

About the Authors

Coach Steve Sperry:

Steve is the owner of Inventive Dental Solutions. He has been a dental advisor providing dental-specific coaching, consulting, and team building for over 25 years. In 1987, Steve fulfilled his lifelong dream of owning his own company and founded Pinnacle Practices, Inc., which grew into the largest dental consulting firm in the South. Over 18 years, Steve developed in-house programs, teaching strategies, and workshops for his dental clients and worked "hands-on" with over 5000 dental teams, ensuring their success and happiness. In addition, Steve has lectured regularly at dental schools, dental societies, universities, and study groups, and contributed several articles to dental journals and magazines.

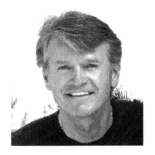

That's what we're doing, changing lives, saving lives.
-Coach Steve Sperry

Visit our Website

for current information, additional tips, tricks, encouragement, and links to our podcast.

HygieneSuperstar.com

Made in the USA
Las Vegas, NV
19 May 2023